Percutaneous and Non-fluoroscopical (PAN) Procedure for Structural Heart Disease

Xiangbin Pan · Ziyad M. Hijazi · Horst Sievert

Percutaneous and Non-fluoroscopical (PAN) Procedure for Structural Heart Disease

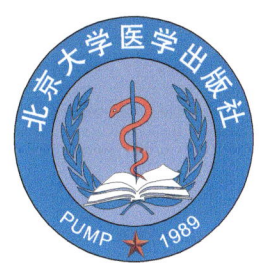

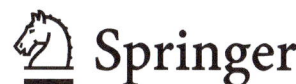

Xiangbin Pan
Structural Heart Disease
Fu Wai Hospital
Beijing
China

Ziyad M. Hijazi
Sidra Medical & Research Center
Doha
Qatar

Horst Sievert
Sankt Katharinen
CardioVascular Center Frankfurt
Frankfurt am Main
Hessen
Germany

ISBN 978-981-15-2054-9   ISBN 978-981-15-2055-6   (eBook)
https://doi.org/10.1007/978-981-15-2055-6

The edition is not for sale in Mainland of China. Customers from Mainland of China please order the print book from:
Peking University Medical Press.

This Springer imprint is published by the registered company Springer Nature Singapore Pte Ltd.
The registered company address is: 152 Beach Road, #21-01/04 Gateway East, Singapore 189721, Singapore

This book is translated from the Chinese version entitled "无放射线经皮介入治疗结构性心脏病" (Percutaneous and Non-fluoroscopical procedure for structural heart disease) published by Peking University Medical Press in 2018. We extend our gratitude to all authors of the original Chinese version:

1. Long Chen: Fuwai Hospital, PUMC&CAMS, Beijing, China;

2. Yao Liu: Fuwai Hospital, PUMC&CAMS, Beijing, China;

3. Wenbin Ouyang: Fuwai Hospital, PUMC&CAMS, Beijing, China;

4. Xiangbin Pan: Fuwai Hospital, PUMC&CAMS, Beijing, China;

5. Kunjing Pang: Fuwai Hospital, PUMC&CAMS, Beijing, China;

6. Shouzheng Wang: Fuwai Hospital, PUMC&CAMS, Beijing, China;

7. Bin Wen: Fuwai Hospital, PUMC&CAMS, Beijing, China;

8. Yongquan Xie: Fuwai Hospital, PUMC&CAMS, Beijing, China;

9. Dawei Zhang: Fuwai Hospital, PUMC&CAMS, Beijing, China;

10. Fengwen Zhang: Fuwai Hospital, PUMC&CAMS, Beijing, China;

11. Li Zhang: Fuwai Hospital, PUMC&CAMS, Beijing, China;

12. Yanbo Zhang: Fuwai Hospital, PUMC&CAMS, Beijing, China;

13. Zhe Zhang: Fuwai Hospital, PUMC&CAMS, Beijing, China;

14. Guangzhi Zhao: Fuwai Hospital, PUMC&CAMS, Beijing, China;

15. Mengxuan Zou: Fuwai Hospital, PUMC&CAMS, Beijing, China.

Foreword

The treatment of structural heart disease, from congenital to valvular, carries the risk of iatro-genic injury from thoracotomy and cardiopulmonary bypass during surgery or radiation and contrast agent use during conventional percutaneous interventional procedures.

Over 10 years of unremitting efforts, Prof. Xiangbin Pan from the National Center of Cardiovascular Disease, Fuwai Hospital, China, developed a percutaneous echocardiography-guided approach for the treatment of atrial and ventricular septal defects, patent ductus arterio-sus, aortic, mitral, and pulmonary stenosis, coarctation of the aorta and atrial fibrillation, among others.

By overcoming the need for a surgical operation room or catheter lab, general anesthesia or tracheal intubation, the cheaper and more accessible non-fluoroscopic approach precludes radiation and contrast agent use, simplifies medical equipment needs, and when advanced from transesophageal to transthoracic can be used on an outpatient basis which renders it par-ticularly suitable to remote areas with insufficient medical resources.

With favorable safety and effectiveness underscored by experience in over 20 developed and developing countries, this approach could potentially be used to treat more complex car-diac malformations. Therefore, with support from the American College of Cardiology (ACC) and the Society for Cardiovascular Angiography and Interventions (SCAI), a group of FACC and MSCAI from the United States, the United Kingdom, France, Canada, Germany, Italy, Turkey, and Japan translated the book entitled *Percutaneous and non-fluoroscopic procedure for structural heart disease* from Chinese to English.

As a summary of valuable multidisciplinary team experiences, this textbook familiarizes cardiologists with basic knowledge, clinical practice considerations, and techniques for percu-taneous echocardiography-guided interventional procedures for various structural heart dis-eases. Aided by videos in every chapter, the book also provides details on working distance, catheter trimming, pulmonary vein deployment technique, and application of novel echo-guided wires, among others, which ease the reader's learning curve.

Shengshou Hu
Fuwai Hospital, PUMC & CAMS; National Center for Cardiovascular Diseases,
Beijing, China
National Clinical Research Center for Cardiovascular Diseases, Beijing, China

Introduction to the Book

The rapid evolution of transcatheter therapies for structural heart disease (SHD) often requires expensive and advanced technology which may be available in only a limited number of academic centers. The lack of trained multidisciplinary specialists in SHD combined with suboptimal technical facilities in many institutions has created an "access-to-care" crisis. This dilemma is accentuated in developing countries, they have the special challenge of managing healthcare for vast numbers of patients in rural locations. Therefore, Chinese physician leaders have been encouraged to develop innovative cost-effective solutions to provide optimal care for a growing number of patients with severe SHD syndromes.

Prof. Xiangbin Pan, from the National Center of Cardiovascular Disease, Fuwai Hospital in China, has authored a novel textbook entitled *Percutaneous and Non-fluoroscopical Procedure for Structural Heart Disease* which was first published in China in 2016 and republished in 2018. In this textbook, Dr. Pan offers what may be an important step forward in the healthcare management of SHD patients by describing in detail the techniques for performing non-fluoroscopic, echocardiographic-guided procedures including: atrial and ventricular septal defect occlusion, patent ductus arteriosus occlusion, transcatheter aortic valve implantation, percutaneous balloon mitral commissurotomy, pulmonary valvuloplasty for pulmonic stenosis, dilatation of coarctation of the aorta, and closure of the left atrial appendage. His novel approach to SHD interventions using echocardiographic guidance without the requirement of fluoroscopic imaging or a conventional catheterization laboratory has the potential to importantly expand accessibility for patients, will significantly decrease economic expenditures, reduce complications associated with iodinated contrast agents, and eliminate exposure of the patient and structural heart team to unnecessary radiation. Transcatheter therapy for SHD is among the fastest growing subspecialties in cardiovascular medicine. An essential component has been multi-modality noninvasive imaging for diagnosis, procedure guidance, and follow-up. Dr. Pan has cultivated a unique skill and makes a strong case to further elevate echo guidance for SHD procedures, as demonstrated clearly in his latest textbook edition. With the supportive contribution from ACC and SCAI, experts from the United States, the United Kingdom, France, Canada, Germany, Italy, Turkey, and Japan for translating the book *Percutaneous and Non-fluroscopical Procedure for Structural Heart Disease* from Chinese to English version.

Although this approach of sole echo guidance may not be optimal for some patients and may gain acceptance initially in more resource-constrained environments, the learned skills will have widespread application in advancing transcatheter SHD treatment. Moreover, the inexorable bond between the proceduralists (surgeons and interventionalists) and imaging experts is strongly reinforced when applying the innovation model of Dr. Pan. For these reasons, we avidly embrace the dissemination of this creative new textbook within the SHD community, as another valued tool which can be incorporated into the SHD treatment armamentarium.

New York-Presbyterian Hospital
Columbia University Medical Center, NY, USA   Rebecca T. Hanh

New York-Presbyterian Hospital
Columbia University Medical Center, NY, USA   Martin B. Leon

Contents

Contributors

Ramazan Akdemir Sakarya University, Sakarya, Turkey

Gianfranco Butera Evelina London Children's Hospital, London, UK

Qiling Cao Rush University Medical Centre, Chicago, IL, USA

Mario Carminati Policlinico San Donato, Milan, Italy

Ruchira Garg Cedars Sinai Medical Center, Los Angeles, CA, USA

Osamu Hashimoto Furano Hospital, Fukuoka, Japan

Ziyad M. Hijazi Sidra Medical & Research Center, Doha, Qatar

Yat-Yin Lam The Chinese University of Hong Kong, Prince of Wales Hospital, Hong Kong, China

Hongxin Li Provincial Hospital Affiliated to Shandong University, Jinan, China

Guitti Milani Necker-Children Diseases Hospital, Paris, France

Joaquim Miró University of MontrealMontreal, QC, Canada

Caroline Ovaert La Timone Hospital, Marseille, France

Xiangbin Pan Fuwai Hospital, PUMC&CAMS, Beijing, China

Shakeel A. Qureshi Evelina London Children's Hospital, London, UK

Mounir Riahi St. Paul's Hospital, Vancouver, BC, Canada

Horst Sievert Cardiovascular Center Frankfurt, Frankfurt, Germany

Jingping Sun Emory University, Atlanta, GA, USA

Evan Zahn Cedars Sinai Medical Center, Los Angeles, CA, USA

Structural heart disease refers to any disease that is related to the abnormal structure of the heart or large vessels and its treatment concept including correcting or changing the structure of the heart. The common types include: (1) congenital heart disease (ventricular septal defect, atrial septal defect, patent ductus arteriosus, etc.), (2) valvular disease (mitral valve, tricuspid valve, aortic valve, and pulmonary valve disease), (3) cardiomyopathy (hypertrophic cardiomyopathy, dilated cardiomyopathy, etc.), (4) abnormal heart structures associated with other diseases (ventricular septal perforation after myocardial infarction or aneurysm).

Structural heart disease occurs in patients from newborns to the seniors, and is a serious threat to life. Congenital heart disease is most common. If not treated in time, it not only seriously affects quality of life, but also can cause fatal complications such as pulmonary arterial hypertension. On the other hand, with the continuous extension of the average life expectancy, degenerative valvular disease is increasingly affecting the lives of senior patients. Conventional surgical and interventional therapies for structural heart disease have advantages and disadvantages, such as avoidance of radiation but huge trauma with long recovery time for the former and minimal trauma but use of fluoroscopy and contrast agents in most patients for the latter. Although their fusion has led to the development and spread of transthoracic instrument closure, which avoids the use of fluoroscopy and contrast agents, differences and debates between disciplines still exist, and proponents of hybrid or percutaneous approaches emphasize their respective advantages. The divergence could be resolved by rapid development of techniques with one that captures the benefits of both treatment approaches while avoiding their pitfalls for instance by utilizing neither conventional surgery nor fluoroscopy, which has proven difficult. Many years ago, we had performed transesophageal echocardiography (TEE)-guided percutaneous closure of atrial septal defect. However, after the initial excitement, only two papers during the ensuing decade reported on experiences with this technique. Why such a good technique had not been applied extensively? The technique is challenging because echocardiography guidance does not always allow catheter localization resulting in procedural failure and serious complications; and tracheal intubation is necessary to prevent suffocation during transesophageal echocardiography guidance. These render TEE-guided percutaneous procedure costlier and more burdensome than fluoroscopic guidance. Therefore, most interventional cardiologists opted for fluoroscopy again.

To foster innovation of effective minimally invasive approaches, a multidisciplinary team focused on hybrid techniques was established at Fuwai Hospital, National Center of Cardiovascular Diseases, China in 2007. Following the principle of "capturing everyone's excellence" and after acquiring sufficient running-in and rich clinical experience, the team spearheaded the development and refinement of echocardiography-guided percutaneous intervention for structural heart disease. At present, percutaneous and Non-fluoroscopical (PAN) procedure for atrial septal defect (ASD), ventricular septal defect (VSD), patent ductus arteriosus (PDA), pulmonary stenosis (PS), coarctation of the aorta (CoA), and atrial fibrillation (AF) can be performed safely and efficaciously at lower cost. More than ten new technologies have been reported for the first time in the world. PAN procedure had progressed from treating only ASD to a wide range of diseases, completing a progression from a single technique to a methodology. Clinical practice with thousands of cases has underscored safety and efficacy of the new percutaneous. The success rate was up to 99% without severe complications, such as cardiac perforation, cardiac tamponade, valve injury, immediate occluder dislodgement and migration or other. Most (more than 95%) of these intervention procedures were guided by the transthoracic echocardiogram (TTE). More importantly, it is a sustainable innovation and we are constantly applying the idea of percutaneous non-fluoroscopy to treat more diseases. However, they are technically challenging with a long learning curve to adjust to its completely different working principle relative to ultrasound and fluoroscopy. Fluoroscopy guidance is based on projections. After X-rays penetrate the three-dimensional human body and device, stereoscopic images are overlapped and displayed as a two-dimensional image, thereby allowing to determine the position and shape of a guide wire. In contrast, ultrasound is based on individual section imaging of three-dimensional objects, providing several two-dimensional images but one section at a time, thereby precluding clear delineation of the entire catheter and guide wire contours to guide them going through the lesion. In order to promote the technology, we have designed special devices for different diseases according to the experience of thousands of patients in clinical practices. With these specially designed devices, it can greatly shorten the learning curve and enable young physicians to carry out these techniques more quickly and safely.

We suggest the following items for PAN percutaneous: (1) A highly experienced team. Operators should be experienced in performing routine percutaneous interventions under fluoroscopy guidance. To maximize safety for patients, interventional procedures should be performed in an operating room in new centers, in case a thoracotomy is needed for cardiac surgery. (2) Marking of working length. Before the procedure, the operator should measure the working length, i.e., the length between a site on chest wall and peripheral vessel puncture site, and mark it on the catheter. When the catheter reaches this length within the body, the tip of catheter should be detected by echocardiogram; we can perform the procedure according to cardiac imaging to avoid inserting catheter too deep to damage the heart. (3) Marking of exchange length. After the guiding catheter aids guide wire crossing through the lesion, the catheter insertion depth should be marked upon its withdrawal as reference for the insertion depth of delivery sheath or balloon catheter. Because body and illness differ among patients, marking this distance individually can effectively avoid untimely guide wire withdrawal before sheath or balloon catheter reaches the lesion and inserting the guide wire too deep causing damage to the heart. (4) Appropriate device selection. Echocardiography only examines one view at a time which renders it difficult to accurately determine catheter and guide wire position. To address the latter limitation, an echocardiography-guided wire can be introduced first; the large size of its tip facilitates guide wire and catheter position detection by echocardiogram. Special catheters, including right coronary and cobra catheters, can be used when entry into the right ventricle through the tricuspid valve is difficult. For patients with PDA and VSD, the pigtail catheter head should be appropriately trimmed to form a 1/2–3/4 arc according to shunt direction, in order to facilitate guide wire passing the lesion. (5) Appropriate patient selection. Because there are

no alike patients, techniques need to be adapted accordingly. In this book, we introduce several techniques for one disease. Every technique has its own advantages and disadvantages. For example, closure by femoral vein approach is preferred for patients with PDA diameter ≥ 5 mm; by femoral artery approach for patients having funnel shaped PDA with diameter at pulmonary artery side <5 mm; by femoral artery approach for patients with distance between VSD and aortic valve ≥ 2 mm, and by jugular vein when distance is ≤ 2 mm. (6) Gradual learning of echocardiography-guided percutaneous interventions. Given its technical difficulty, beginners should gradually advance through the complexity spectrum of echocardiography-guided percutaneous interventions, starting with ASD closure and PDA closure, and then pulmonary valve balloon valvuloplasty and LAA closure, and finally VSD closure and valvuloplasty. TEE guidance should be used firstly and then TTE guidance. TEE images are clearer because the probe is close to the left atrial posterior wall and the heart is in the near field of the ultrasound beam. For patients with thin chest wall, TTE can better display cardiac anatomy and guide catheter and guide wire through the lesion, which is not the case for patients with thick chest wall, which limits ultrasound wave penetration leading to failed closure.

PAN procedure not only protect patients from pain and other complications associated with conventional surgery, but also obviate the use of fluoroscopy or contrast agents. This avoids risk of radiation damage, allergy, and renal function impairment, hence potentially increases clinical use. In the process of exploration, we overcome technical difficulties, change transesophageal echocardiography to transthoracic echocardiography, avoid general anesthesia, endotracheal intubation, and achieve "no scalpel, no radiation, no tracheal intubation" to treat structural heart disease. The approach requires commonly ultrasound devices, not expensive radiographic ones, rendering it cheaper and safer. PAN procedure had been performed in out-patient department to save more patients and medical cost, it is more ideal for hospitals with limited infrastructure and capabilities. More importantly, because cumulative radiation damage may greatly increase cancer risk, the approach is not only beneficial to patients but also to medical personnel who are exposed to radiation for thousands of minutes yearly. Therefore, echocardiography-guided percutaneous interventions free overworked medical staff from having to wear the heavy and uncomfortably warm lead protectors required in fluoroscopy procedure and are broadly to treat a growing spectrum of diseases.

In both developed countries emphasizing iatrogenic injury reduce and pursuing quality improvement, and developing countries with relative poor medical conditions and a large number of patients to be treated, echocardiography-guided percutaneous intervention has been applied well. Colleagues from more than 30 countries and regions around the world, including the France, Italy, Japan, Kenya, Russia, Turkey, Ukraine, United Kingdom and United States, come to Fuwai hospital to learn this new technique. We are using these techniques to save more lives in more countries. Although some experts believe that the traditional techniques of using radiation are better, and even think that the harm of radiation is "not enough to worry about," they still wear lead clothes to protect themselves when they are performing the procedure, and patients still have to be exposed to radiation. Controversy is meaningless, because advances in technology rely on strength rather than argument. In the following chapters, we will take you through the advantages of this technology and once again prove the universal law of survival of the fittest: we can do it and hope to help you can also do it. The great advantages of "protecting patients and doctors, lowering costs" have given us a good clinical application prospect of PAN procedure. Now, let us begin to help more people!

Echocardiography-guided percutaneous interventions for structural heart disease can be carried out in normal operating rooms, hybrid operating rooms, or catheter laboratories meeting infection control criteria. In order to facilitate the smooth progress of interventions, sedation or general anesthesia is required for patients, to relieve their discomfort or pain during percutaneous interventions. Safe and efficacious peri-procedural management of anesthesia requires anesthesiologists, who have mastered anesthetic techniques in both children and adults, because the patients involved can be either children or adults. Since the procedure may have to be converted into minimally invasive surgery or traditional cardiovascular surgery with cardiopulmonary bypass, trained cardiac anesthesiologists, who are familiar with the pathophysiology of structural heart disease and procedural details of intervention, are required. In addition, it is the responsibility of the anesthesiologists to monitor and maintain stable vital signs of patients. Ideal anesthesia management translates to post-intervention transfer of patients in the best possible status to regular wards or intensive care units.

2.1 Preparations Before Anesthesia

Compared with traditional cardiovascular surgery, echocardiography-guided percutaneous interventions for structural heart disease have obvious technical advantages. However, these procedures are not without potential risks. By providing the best possible pre-anesthetic preparations, anesthesiologists can contribute maximally to reduce potential peri-procedural risks.

2.1.1 Pre-anesthetic Visit

Visiting patients before anesthesia and interventional therapy is important and necessary for anesthesiologists to estab-

lish a rapport and mutual trust with patients and their families; evaluate patients' overall status; obtain signatures on relevant medical documents; and communicate with interventionalists about interventional therapy plans.

- Psychological preparation before anesthesia is important, particularly for patients undergoing interventions under local anesthesia plus mild sedation. If the patient is an adult, direct communication can ease tension and anxiety; if the patient is a small child, there should be sufficient communication with the family as well to obtain their trust and cooperation.
- Past history of surgery, anesthesia, and allergy should be documented in detail. Comorbidities (including hypertension, diabetes, coronary heart disease, and arrhythmia) should be appropriately managed. In addition to observing the patient's general condition, physical examination should focus on cardiopulmonary auscultation, blood pressure measurement of bilateral upper and lower extremities, and evaluation of difficult airways. In some children, evaluation of development and intelligence should be carried out. Relevant cardiac testing (including electrocardiography, chest radiography, and echocardiography) and laboratory evaluation (including blood gas analysis, basic hematology and biochemical panels, coagulation function, and infectious disease tests) are necessary to evaluate vital organ function. Drugs in use should be reconfirmed to judge whether these drugs should be continued or stopped. If patients have increased risks of peri-procedural complications (e.g., upper respiratory tract infection with body temperature above 38 °C and increased leukocyte count), pertinent treatment should be instituted first, interventional therapy delayed if necessary.
- In order to formulate individualized anesthesia program, anesthesiologists should communicate with interventionalists to understand challenges of the interventional therapy plan and its anesthesia management requirements.

© Peking University Medical Press 2020
X. Pan et al., *Percutaneous and Non-fluoroscopical (PAN) Procedure for Structural Heart Disease*,
https://doi.org/10.1007/978-981-15-2055-6_2

- For patients at risk of pre-procedural anemia or peri-procedural bleeding, red blood cells, fresh frozen plasma, or platelet concentrate should be available.
- Medical documents associated with anesthesia should be signed in keeping with the law and hospital policy. The anesthesiologists should keep the patients and their families informed of the anesthesia plan and the potential risks. An informed consent form for anesthesia should be signed after patients and families fully understand relevant anesthetic details and risks of anesthesia.

2.1.2 Pre-anesthetic Fasting

All patients receiving echocardiography-guided percutaneous interventions for structural heart disease must fast before anesthesia to avoid regurgitation and aspiration during the procedure.

- Fasting requirements are age driven. Children have vigorous metabolic activity with rapid liquid loss, which makes them more prone to dehydration and metabolic acidosis; therefore, the younger the patient, the shorter the fasting period. The detailed fasting plan should be formulated taking into consideration the relative guidelines, routines established in local institutions, and comorbidities (e.g., diabetes).
- If anesthesia cannot start on time, water, dextrose, and electrolytes can be given parenterally to adults or children to avoid internal environment disorders.

2.1.3 Pre-anesthetic Medication

Pre-anesthetic medications aim to relieve tension and anxiety in patients, inhibit secretion in salivary and mucous glands and reduce the untoward effects of excessive adrenaline secretion in some diseases (e.g., cardiac valve stenosis).

- There exists no common practice in pre-anesthetic medications. The type, dose, and route of administration of pre-anesthetic medications vary among individuals. Anticholinergics and sedatives are the most common drugs, which can be administrated intramuscularly or intravenously. Atropine and midazolam are commonly used.
- For infants, the elderly, pregnant women, or patients with concomitant diseases, pre-anesthetic medication should be carefully selected according to clinical needs before interventional therapy. If there is a clear contraindication of medication, no pre-anesthetic drug will be given.

2.1.4 Anesthesia Monitoring (Fig. 2.1) and Anesthetic Drugs

Anesthesiologists should use appropriate anesthesia monitoring devices and anesthetic drugs in different circumstances in order to ensure that interventional therapy will be carried out successfully and safely. Expensive anesthesia monitoring devices or anesthetic drugs cannot reduce the incidence of complications; it is the advanced management of anesthesia that plays the most important role in the safety of patients during interventional procedures. Therefore, anesthesiologists should use anesthesia monitoring devices and anesthetic drugs individually during interventional procedures to evaluate and maintain the vital signs of patients and be responsible for their selection to ensure the lowest medical cost based on medical safety. Anesthesia monitoring can be noninvasive or invasive, and their benefit-risk ratio should be considered.

- Electrocardiography (ECG), arterial blood pressure, and pulse oxygen saturation are basic monitoring items that must be used in echocardiography-guided percutaneous interventions for structural heart disease. Electrocardiography is used to monitor the heart's electrical activity to detect arrhythmias, heart conduction blocks and myocardial ischemia that could be secondary to blood electrolyte imbalances, and use of anesthetics, vasoactive agents, and interventional devices, during

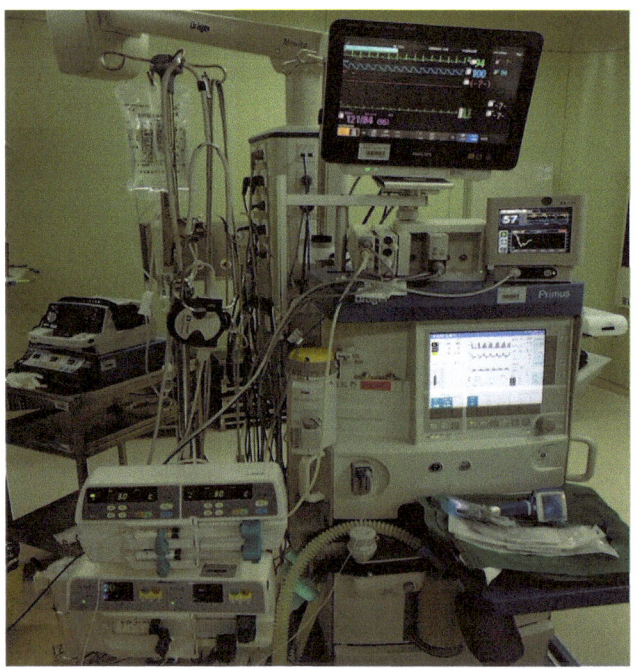

Fig. 2.1 Real scene of anesthesia monitoring

interventional procedures. Arterial blood pressure is the basic monitoring index to assess blood supply to organs and tissues reflecting cardiovascular status. Arterial blood pressure can be obtained by indirect noninvasive or direct invasive measurement. For most patients, non-invasive blood pressure monitoring with the automatic oscillography technique (the belt electronic pressure measuring device) can be used during interventional procedure. However, invasive arterial blood pressure monitoring could be the preferred technique in balloon valvuloplasty for valvular stenosis in some patients. Pulse oxygen saturation is a basic monitoring index to assist in observing the oxygenation status of the patient during interventional therapy. During anesthesia, pulse oxygen saturation of patients should not be less than 95%. Because the pulse oxygen saturation does not reflect the use of oxygen in the tissue, blood gas analysis should be performed if necessary.

- For patients receiving general anesthesia with mechanical ventilation or spontaneous breathing, ventilation status is continuously and noninvasively monitored by following the concentration or partial pressure of carbon dioxide in expired air. This index can also reflect hemodynamic changes in pulmonary circulation and systemic circulation. Common reasons for a sudden decrease in carbon dioxide in expiratory air include: air leakage or blockage of the respiratory tract, abnormal pulmonary ventilation or gas exchange function, and reduced cardiac output.

- The relatively large body surface area and incomplete thermoregulation in infants places them at a high risk of low body temperatures during interventional therapy, which may increase myocardial oxygen consumption, induce arrhythmias and affect coagulation function. Core temperature measured as nasopharyngeal, rectal, or bladder temperature is always required during long interventional therapies, especially for infants with low body weight. To avoid low body temperatures, it is imperative to improve the environmental temperature and recommend a heated mattress in accordance with monitoring information. Also, fluids for intravenous infusion and inhaled air should be properly heated, especially for infants. In addition, temperature monitoring is indispensable for patients at risk of malignant hyperthermia.

- Bispectral index (BIS) monitoring, a derivative of electroencephalography, assesses a patient's consciousness status and anesthesia depth, assisting the anesthesiologist in better implementing "fast-track" cardiac anesthesia and reducing the incidence of awareness in general anesthesia patients. However, it is important to realize that BIS monitoring cannot predict movement of extremity caused by pain stimulation.

- Anesthetic medications should be prepared in accordance with the hospital's drug reserve and prescribing habits of anesthesiologists, including sedatives, analgesics, and neuromuscular blocking agents. As unforeseen circumstances might endanger a patient's life during percutaneous intervention, the operating room or the catheter laboratory should be equipped for resuscitation with dextrose injection, atropine, epinephrine, norepinephrine, dopamine, isoproterenol, calcium chloride or calcium gluconate, sodium bicarbonate, lidocaine, corticosteroids, and aminophylline, among others.

2.2 Management of Anesthesia

The aim of anesthesia management during echocardiography-guided percutaneous interventions for structural heart disease is to keep patients relaxed and pain-free with stable ventilation and circulation. Addressing variations in degree of cooperation and pain tolerance of patients and procedural duration requires cooperation among doctors from multiple departments (including interventionalists, anesthesiologists, sonographers, and surgeons). Therefore, the anesthesiologist should customize type of anesthesia (Table 2.1) and anesthetic agent use (Table 2.2) according to age, illness degree, complexity of interventional therapy, and procedural demands by doctors from different departments.

Types of anesthesia include local anesthesia plus sedation and general anesthesia. Local anesthesia plus sedation, which is suitable for adults or children who can cooperate during interventional therapies, allows the anesthesiologist to manage pain and discomfort, maintain satisfactory respiratory and circulatory functions, and allows patients to respond to verbal instructions from interventionalists, anesthesiologists, or sonographers. With general anesthesia, spontaneous breathing can be preserved, while mechanical ventilation can be used when needed. General anesthesia with tracheal intubation is used if the interventional procedure is converted to surgery because of technical difficulties. Mechanical ventilation may cause changes in hemodynamics, and therefore general anesthesia which preserves spontaneous breathing is preferred.

After confirming the type of anesthesia, the anesthesiologist should choose the appropriate anesthetic agent based on the evaluation of patients. The specific dose of anesthetic agents should be determined based on the experience of local medical institutions.

Table 2.1 Preferred types of anesthesia in Fuwai Hospital (for reference only)

Interventional therapy		Local anesthesia plus sedation	General anesthesia (spontaneous breathing)	General anesthesia (mechanical ventilation)
PDA closure	Adult	√	√	
	Child	√	√	
ASD closure	Adult	√	√	
	Child	√	√	
VSD closure	Adult	√	√	
	Child	√	√	
Balloon valvuloplasty for pulmonary valve stenosis	Adult	√	√	
	Child	√	√	
Balloon valvuloplasty for mitral valve stenosis	Adult	√	√	
Balloon valvuloplasty for aortic valve stenosis	Adult		√	√
	Child			√
Left atrial appendage occlusion	Adult		√	√
Stent implantation for coarctation of aorta	Adult		√	√
	Child		√	√

Table 2.2 Anesthetic agents commonly used in Fuwai Hospital (for reference only)

Anesthetics	Induction	Maintenance
Midazolam	0.1–0.15 mg/kg	0.05–0.1 mg/(kg·h)
Propofol	1–2 mg/kg	2–5 mg/(kg·h)
Ketamine	0.5–2 mg/kg	1–2 mg/(kg·h)
Dexmedetomidine	0.5–1 μg/kg	0.2–1.4 μg/(kg·h)
Sevoflurane	3–4%	1–2%
Fentanyl	0.5–8 μg/kg	0.5–5 μg/(kg·h)
Sufentanil	0.1–1 μg/kg	0.1–0.5 μg/(kg·h)
Cisatracurium	0.1–0.3 mg/kg	0.1–0.3 mg/(kg·h)

2.2.1 Anesthesia Management in Echocardiography-Guided Interventional Therapy for Septal Defect and Patent Ductus Arteriosus

So far, echocardiography-guided interventional therapy can be carried out in various types of congenital heart defects (CHD), including atrial septal defect (ASD), ventricular septal defect (VSD), and patent ductus arteriosus (PDA). Local anesthesia plus sedation or general anesthesia with spontaneous breathing is the preferred type of anesthesia in patients for interventional therapy guided by transthoracic echocardiography (TTE).

• Upon arrival in the operating room or the catheter laboratory, patients should be placed under monitoring for electrocardiography, arterial blood pressure, and pulse oxygen saturation. A peripheral vein line should be established for anesthetic agent administration and liquid supplementation. Noninvasive blood pressure should be measured in a limb different from that with the peripheral vein line. The depth of anesthesia can be determined according to the patient's response to painful stimuli in

patients under local anesthesia plus sedation. However, BIS monitoring is recommended for patients under general anesthesia.

• Anesthetics for anesthesia induction and maintenance include midazolam, propofol, ketamine, dexmedetomidine, sevoflurane, fentanyl, and sufentanil. During the procedure, patients are supplied with oxygen delivered through face masks. During anesthesia management, an increased dose of ketamine or dexmedetomidine can provide a satisfactory effect in little children with body movement due to intolerance to pain. Anesthesiologists should decide the dosage of anesthetics and the timing of withdrawal according to the process of interventional therapy. If there are no complications, patients can be transferred directly to a regular ward.

• The typical hemodynamic feature of ASD is a left-to-right atrial shunt. Defect closure can be achieved by deployment of a closure device via the femoral or jugular vein. With satisfactory hemodynamics, infusion rate should not be too fast after successful closure of ASD, to avoid excessive cardiac preload leading to acute left ventricular dysfunction.

• The typical hemodynamic feature of VSD is a left-to-right ventricular shunt. Defect closure can be accomplished by deployment of a closure device via the femoral artery or jugular vein. Echocardiography-guided VSD closure is technically challenging and requires a longer procedural time. Therefore, it is a better choice to intubate with a laryngeal mask in little children under general anesthesia with spontaneous breathing to facilitate the monitoring of exhaled carbon dioxide and the use of volatile anesthetics (e.g., sevoflurane). Anesthesiologists should pay close attention to patients' rhythm changes because of possible endocardial stimulation by the catheter or guide wire.

- The typical hemodynamic feature of PDA is an aorta to pulmonary artery shunt. Abnormal blood flow between aorta and pulmonary artery can be blocked by feeding occluder into arterial duct through femoral artery or femoral vein. During the procedure, arterial blood pressure should be measured in both upper and lower extremities to detect any blockage of the descending aorta caused by the occluder. With the right lower extremity preferred by interventionalists for the procedure, the right upper limb and the left lower extremity are preferred for invasive or noninvasive blood pressure monitoring. When releasing the occluder, controlled hypotension is induced as needed. Sodium nitroprusside can be administered intravenously at 0.6 μg/(kg·min) initially, and the infusion rate should be adjusted according to the patient's blood pressure. During controlled hypotension, attention should be paid to ECG and pulse oxygen saturation changes reflecting myocardial and peripheral tissue perfusion changes.

2.2.2   Anesthesia Management in Echocardiography-Guided Interventional Therapy for Valvular Heart Diseases

In Fuwai Hospital, echocardiography-guided percutaneous interventions can be carried out in various types of valvular heart diseases, including pulmonary valve stenosis, mitral valve stenosis, and aortic valve stenosis. Most of the procedures can be completed through TTE guidance, among which local anesthesia plus sedation or general anesthesia with spontaneous breathing is preferred. However, general anesthesia with mechanical ventilation is preferred for balloon valvuloplasty for some patients with aortic valve stenosis.

- The anesthesia monitoring and anesthetic drugs in local anesthesia plus sedation or general anesthesia with spontaneous breathing are referred to in "Anesthesia management in echocardiography-guided interventional therapy for septal defect and patent ductus arteriosus."
- Most of the patients who undergo pulmonary valve balloon valvuloplasty are children, while the majority of patients undergoing mitral valve balloon valvuloplasty are adults. Once the balloon is inflated within pulmonary or mitral orifice, blood flow from the right ventricle to the pulmonary artery or from the left atrium to the left ventricle will be temporarily blocked, causing transient decreases in heart rate, arterial blood pressure, or pulse oxygen saturation. Therefore, invasive arterial blood pressure monitoring is recommended if necessary, and availability of prepared vasoactive agents able to improve the heart rate and blood pressure is impor-

tant. Anesthesiologists should make patients inhale oxygen before balloon is inflated to ensure adequate oxygen reservation.
- Prior to inflating the balloon within aortic orifice, the hemodynamic state is usually unstable due to rapid pacing with temporary pacemakers. Therefore, general anesthesia may be supplemented with mechanical ventilation via an endotracheal tube or laryngeal mask in certain patients. Under the circumstances, a central venous access (the right internal jugular vein is most commonly used) is recommended for the implantation of pacing leads and use of vasoactive agents, in addition to continuous invasive arterial blood pressure monitoring.

2.2.3   Anesthesia Management in Echocardiography-Guided Percutaneous Left Atrial Appendage Occlusion and Aortic Stent Implantation

In Fuwai Hospital, echocardiography-guided interventional therapies also include left atrial appendage occlusion and aortic stent implantation, for which TTE is inadequate for clear images. Therefore, transesophageal echocardiography (TEE) guidance is common in these procedures.

- The clinical application of echocardiography-guided percutaneous left atrial appendage occlusion and aortic stent implantation is still in its infancy. In order to ensure the smooth progress of treatments and the comfort and safety of patients, general anesthesia is recommended.
- Left atrial appendage occlusion is a treatment strategy to reduce the risk of thromboembolic events in patients with non valvular atrial fibrillation (AF). Atrial fibrillation with rapid ventricular response may occur in patients undergoing left atrial appendage occlusion during interventional therapy. Therefore, attention should be paid to arrhythmic monitoring, and antiarrhythmic agents and vasoactive agents should be prepared in advance. Due to the long duration of procedure, attention should also be paid to maintaining the stability of patients' internal environment for those patients who undergo left atrial appendage occlusion and septal defect closure simultaneously.
- Echocardiography-guided percutaneous aortic stenting is a treatment approach for coarctation of aorta in adults or adolescents. During the procedure, the arterial blood pressure should be monitored in both upper and lower extremities so as to evaluate the effect of stenting immediately. If controlled hypotension is required, the treatment scheme can be referred to in "Anesthesia management in echocardiography-guided interventional therapy for septal defect and patent ductus arteriosus."

2.2.4 Infection Control and Anticoagulation

In anesthesia management during echocardiography-guided percutaneous interventions for structural heart disease, anesthesiologists should also be responsible for peri-anesthesia infection control and intra-procedural anticoagulation. It is necessary for anesthesiologists to be familiar with infection control measures and grasp the anticoagulation regimen.

- Because nosocomial infections are associated with increased cost and mortality, the quality of peri-anesthesia infection control directly affects the clinical outcomes and prognosis of patients. Infection control measures aim to prevent bacteria from invading the body and to use prophylactic antibiotics. Specific measures to prevent bacteria from invading patients are related to patients, doctors, and the environment in the operating room or the catheter laboratory and should be implemented in accordance with the regulations of local medical institutions. The selection and regimen of prophylactic antibiotics should also be carried out in accordance with the regulations of local medical institutions (Table 2.3).
- Heparin is commonly used to prevent thrombosis in percutaneous interventional therapy. Heparin should be administered intravenously (80–100 U/kg in Fuwai Hospital, excluding PDA closure) after successful vessel puncture. Because of large inter-individual variation, activated clotting time (ACT), 5 min after heparin administration, can be used to assess the effect of anticoagulation. The value of ACT is recommended to be maintained at 200 s or higher, and additional heparin should be administered if ACT falls below the prescribed threshold. After procedures, it is common for most patients not to neutralize anticoagulation effect of heparin. Protamine by intravenous infusion can be used to rapidly antagonize the effects of heparin if necessary. As adverse reactions or side effects of protamine may occur in some patients, anesthesiologists should be familiar with the management measures.

2.2.5 Management of Acute Pain After Echocardiography-Guided Percutaneous Interventional Therapy

Appropriate sedation and analgesia should be performed if the patient has obvious discomfort or pain in the early post-procedure period, in order to relieve discomfort and pain, and avoid bleeding at the puncture site or migration of the occluder device due to moving restlessly.

- Post-procedure pain treatment is usually not required in adults, while sedation may be required.
- Some children may receive post-procedural sedation and analgesia, namely dexmedetomidine and sufentanil.
- During the treatment of post-procedural acute pain, heart rate, arterial blood pressure, and pulse oxygen saturation of patients should be monitored.

2.2.6 Challenges in Anesthesia

It is essential for anesthesiologists to be qualified with the ability to cope with the conversion of anesthesia types and anesthesia-related complications during echocardiography-guided percutaneous interventional therapies.

- Any echocardiography-guided percutaneous intervention has the possibility of being converted to traditional cardiothoracic surgery because of technical difficulties during therapy or unexpected therapeutic results. In such cases, anesthesiologists should achieve a smooth conversion between different types of anesthesia, and invasive arterial blood pressure monitoring and central venous access need to be established quickly if there is a medical emergency. Anesthesiologists should also adjust the dosage of anesthetics according to the changed anesthesia type in order to maintain the stability of patients' vital signs and ensure the smooth progress of surgery.
- If TTE is inadequate for clear images in a few obese patients or in patients with morbidities (e.g., emphysema or thoracic deformity), interventionalists will switch from TTE guidance to TEE guidance during procedure. In order to ensure the smooth progress of percutaneous interventions and the comfort and safety of patients, general anesthesia is recommended.
- With advances of anesthesia technology, anesthesia-related complications during echocardiography-guided percutaneous interventional therapies are rare. Anesthesiologists should still be alert to malignant hyperthermia which is one of the most serious complica-

Table 2.3 Prophylactic antibiotics in Fuwai Hospital (for reference only)

Constitution	Antibiotic	Adult	Child	First administration
Standard	Cefuroxime	1.5 g	20 mg/kg	30–60 min before procedure
Allergic	Clindamycin	0.6 g	10 mg/kg	30–60 min before procedure

tions of anesthesia. Body temperature and exhaled carbon dioxide should be closely monitored in patients at potential risk of malignant hyperthermia. Once malignant hyperthermia is considered, emergency medical procedures approved by local medical institutions should be initiated immediately.

2.3 Prevention and Treatment of Complications Associated with Interventional Therapy

Anesthesiologists should not only prevent and treat anesthesia-related complications, but also actively participate in the prevention and treatment of complications related to interventional procedures. Most complications related to interventional procedures are self-limited; however, timely treatment of severe complications usually requires a cardiac surgeon, who should be on standby during technically complex or high-risk interventional procedures.

2.3.1 Arrhythmia

Direct endocardial stimulation by catheter or guide wire may trigger atrial or ventricular arrhythmias. In cases with single atrial or ventricular premature contractions, interventional procedures can continue without treatment. For ventricular tachycardia, multifocal premature ventricular contractions, or third-degree atrioventricular block, among others, interventionalists must be notified to suspend the procedure to avoid ventricular fibrillation or cardiac arrest. While eliminating mechanical stimulation, circulation and breathing should be closely monitored. If ventricular fibrillation or cardiac arrest happens, cardiopulmonary resuscitation (including cardioversion, external chest compression, and controlled ventilation) must be implemented immediately. If arrhythmia occurs after the end of interventional occlusion, echocardiography should be performed immediately to determine whether if the occluder device migrates.

2.3.2 Valvular Regurgitation

Mild regurgitation may occur after balloon valvuloplasty. Acute valvular regurgitation usually develops instantaneously upon the passage of a catheter or guide wire through the orifice, and valvular regurgitation can disappear spontaneously with the withdrawal of the catheter or guide wire. If the valvular regurgitation happens after the occluder is released, interventionalists should consider other types of occluder or cardiothoracic surgery.

2.3.3 Hypotension

Hypotension may be observed during procedure. Before treatment, the causes of hypotension should be confirmed:

- If hypotension is secondary to arrhythmia, controlling it may resolve the hypotension.
- In children, prolonged fasting may cause acidosis and hypotension. If hypotension is present before interventional therapy, physiological saline with glucose and electrolytes can be given intravenously.
- Errhysis at the catheter's near-end and puncture site may not greatly affect adults. However, during long procedures, blood loss may cause hypotension in children due to hypovolemia.
- Rarely, forceful interventional manipulation may lead to vessel or cardiac perforation with ensuing cardiac tamponade, manifesting as severe hypotension. For patients with persistent massive bleeding, surgery must be carried out as soon as possible.

2.3.4 Cardiac Insufficiency

For patients with cardiac decompensation, acute cardiac insufficiency may develop by excessive mental stress, arrhythmia, and excessive infusion during procedure. Therapeutic principles include elimination of inducing factors, sedation, and administration of cardiotonics, diuretics and vasodilators.

2.3.5 Hypoxic Spells

Patients with pulmonary stenosis may have varying degrees of obstruction of right ventricular outflow tract. Hypoxic spells may occur while a catheter or guide wire passes through the right ventricular outflow tract. The clinical manifestations include rapid decrease of exhaled carbon dioxide, oxygen saturation, and arterial blood pressure. Tachycardia and hypotension during procedures should be avoided in patients with a history of hypoxic spells. During an anoxic attack, high concentration oxygen should be inhaled and depth of anesthesia must be ensured. Vasopressors should be administered if severe drop in blood pressure occurs. Moreover, cardiotonics should be administered if acute cardiac insufficiency occurs.

2.3.6 Pharyngeal and Esophageal Injury

Pharyngeal and esophageal injury is associated with TEE used in interventional therapy. If the TEE probe is difficult to insert, it may cause pharyngeal injury due to repeated attempts or overexertion. Mechanical stimulation produced by the movement of TEE probe and high temperature generated at the distal end of TEE probe may cause esophageal injury.

2.3.7 Thrombosis

The occurrence of thrombosis inside blood vessels after echocardiography-guided percutaneous interventional therapy is very rare and is generally related to patients' own risk factor of hypercoagulability or inappropriate anticoagulation during procedure. Once thrombosis is diagnosed, heparin or thrombolysis can be administered; the need for vascular surgeon is very rare.

3.1 General Considerations

3.1.1 Overview

Two-dimensional (2D) echocardiography, the real-time cardiac imaging technique, is based on ultrasound wave scanning of different points using various views to obtain 2D images of any cardiac cross section. Noninvasiveness, convenience, and lower cost of 2D echocardiography have rendered it first-line tool for heart disease diagnosis; its improved image resolution allows detecting a 2 mm defect in continuous segments of atrial or ventricular septum.

There are three modalities of Doppler echocardiography: pulse wave (PW), which displays real-time blood flow velocity and direction at the point monitored; continuous wave (CW), which by showing continuous transmission pulse wave allows to measure any high-velocity blood flow in the sampling line; and color flow mapping (CFM), which by overlapping blood flow in color to black-and-white 2D or M-type echocardiogram allows to visualize the structural abnormality and associated hemodynamic abnormalities.

3.1.2 Transthoracic Echocardiography (TTE)

A standard transthoracic echocardiogram includes five TTE windows, each providing one or more views of the heart. The right parasternal window is optional and can be used when other views are suboptimal or when additional information is needed:

3.1.2.1 Left Parasternal Window

1. The parasternal long-axis view (Fig. 3.1) shows the left ventricle long axis, left ventricular outflow tract, left atrium, aortic valve, interventricular septum, and bicuspid valve. In this most common cardiac transection, all left ventricular parameters can be quantitated using M-mode with the cursor placed just distal to the mitral valve leaflet tips to measure LV wall thickness and cavity size, as an alternative to 2D measurement, and ejection fraction can be calculated (Fig. 3.2).
2. Parasternal short-axis view (Fig. 3.2): By scanning the heart from base to apex, short-axis views are displayed at successive levels, namely short axis of great arteries around aorta, mitral valve level in left ventricle, papillary muscle level, and cardiac apex level.

3.1.2.2 Apical Window

The apical window includes four- (Fig. 3.3), five-, and two-chamber views, which are optimal for determining ratio and inflow tract of cardiac cavity, and atrioventricular valve position and shape.

3.1.2.3 Subcostal Window

The subcostal window is a better choice for the patient with poor parasternal window, the interatrial septum structure cannot be clearly displayed, and a satisfactory image can be obtained in subcostal view. This view shows the relationship between positions of viscera and heart. The upper and lower vena cava and their connection to the atria can be clearly displayed. In particular, the subcostal double-atrial view is the best cut surface for observing the interatrial septum.

3.1.2.4 Superior Sternum Window

Placing the probe on the suprasternal fossa, the long axis includes the aortic arch and its branches and cross section of right pulmonary artery. This section displays the long-axis image of patent ductus arteriosus.

3.1.3 Transesophageal Echocardiography (TEE)

TTE may not be sensitive enough for diagnosis of patients with acoustic window limitations, such as in thoracic cavity deformity, emphysema, and obesity. Interference by sternum or emphysema in obtaining a clear cardiac image can be avoided

© Peking University Medical Press 2020
X. Pan et al., *Percutaneous and Non-fluoroscopical (PAN) Procedure for Structural Heart Disease*,
https://doi.org/10.1007/978-981-15-2055-6_3

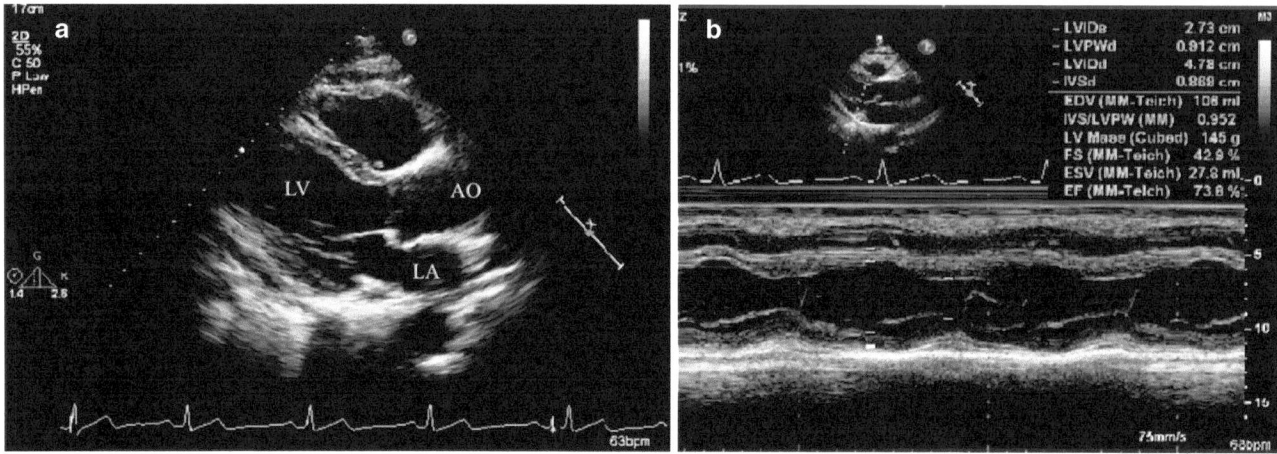

Fig. 3.1 TTE-parasternal long-axis view: (**a**) 2D normal parasternal long-axis view. (**b**) M-mode recording of left ventricle long axis for measurements of left ventricular internal end-diastolic (LVIDd) and end-systolic (LVDs) diameter, interventricular septal end diastolic (LVIDd) and end-systolic (IVSd) thickness, left ventricular posterior wall end diastolic (LVPWd), and end-systolic wall thickness. Calculate left ventricular short-axis fraction shortening (FS) and left ventricular ejection fraction (EF)

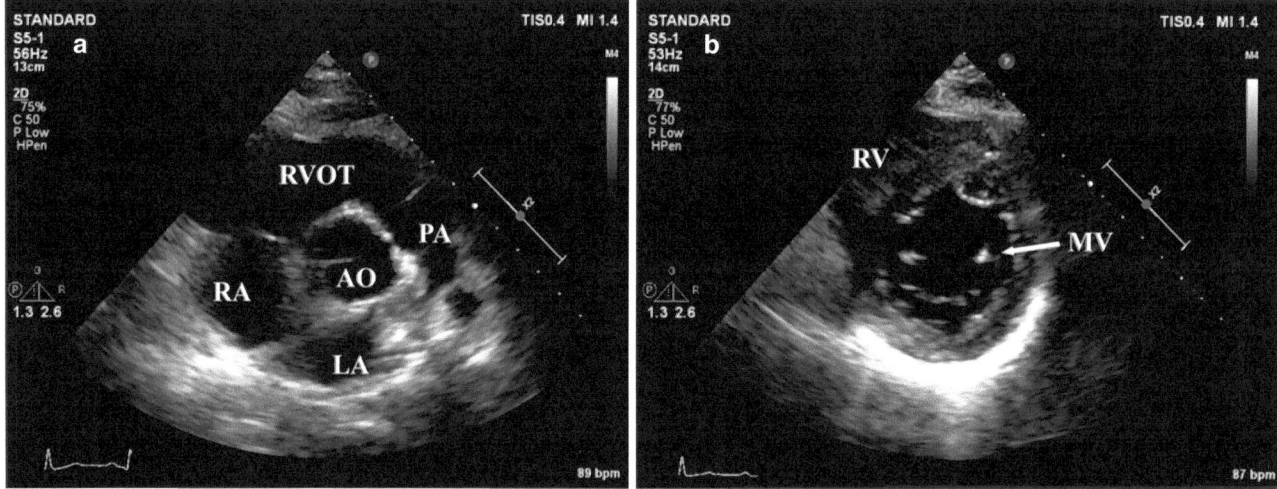

Fig. 3.2 TTE-parasternal short-axis view: (**a**) Normal parasternal short-axis view of great arteries level. (**b**) Left ventricular parasternal short-axis view at mitral valve (↑) level

Fig. 3.3 TTE-apical four-chamber view showed the 2D measurement of the left ventricle

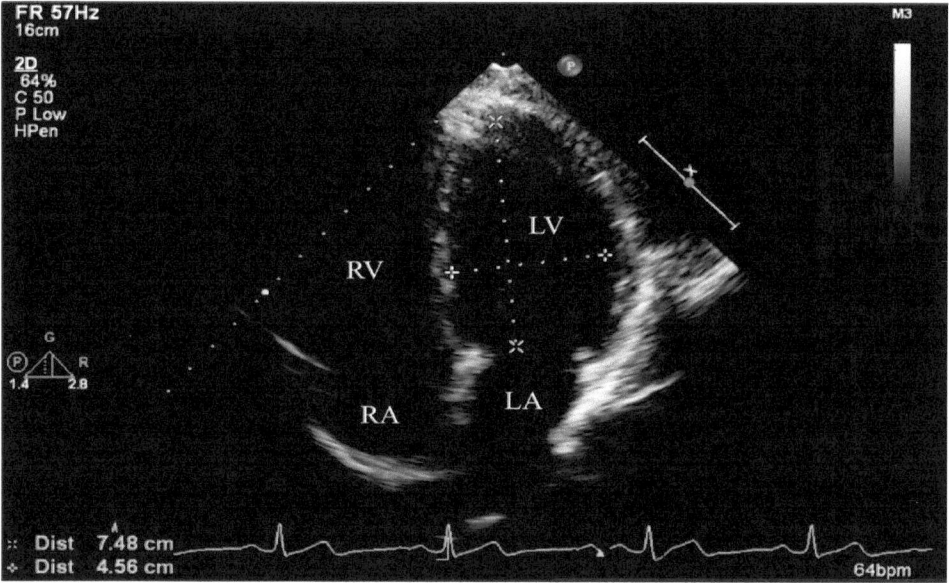

by placing the ultrasound probe in the esophagus which is near the heart. While imaging of atrial septum, left atrial appendage, mitral valve, and aortic valve structure is obviously superior with TEE than TTE, but the aortic arch, pulmonary artery branch, and arterial duct cannot be visualized.

3.1.3.1 TEE Examination

Probe placement in the esophagus is invasive and should be performed in the appropriate rescue setting. Probe should be positioned first in the middle to lower esophagus at the left atrial level for cardiac chamber examination, and then moved up and down to maximize observation field. Because it is easy to cause esophageal mucosal damage, probe insertion and movement should be gentle. The direction of the esophageal probe should be adjusted in case of resistance; the probe should not be inserted forcibly.

3.1.3.2 TEE Standard Views (Fig. 3.4)

3.1.4 Value of Echocardiography in Percutaneous Interventional Therapy for Congenital Heart Disease

Echocardiography has been an indispensable and important monitoring tool since the inception of percutaneous inter-

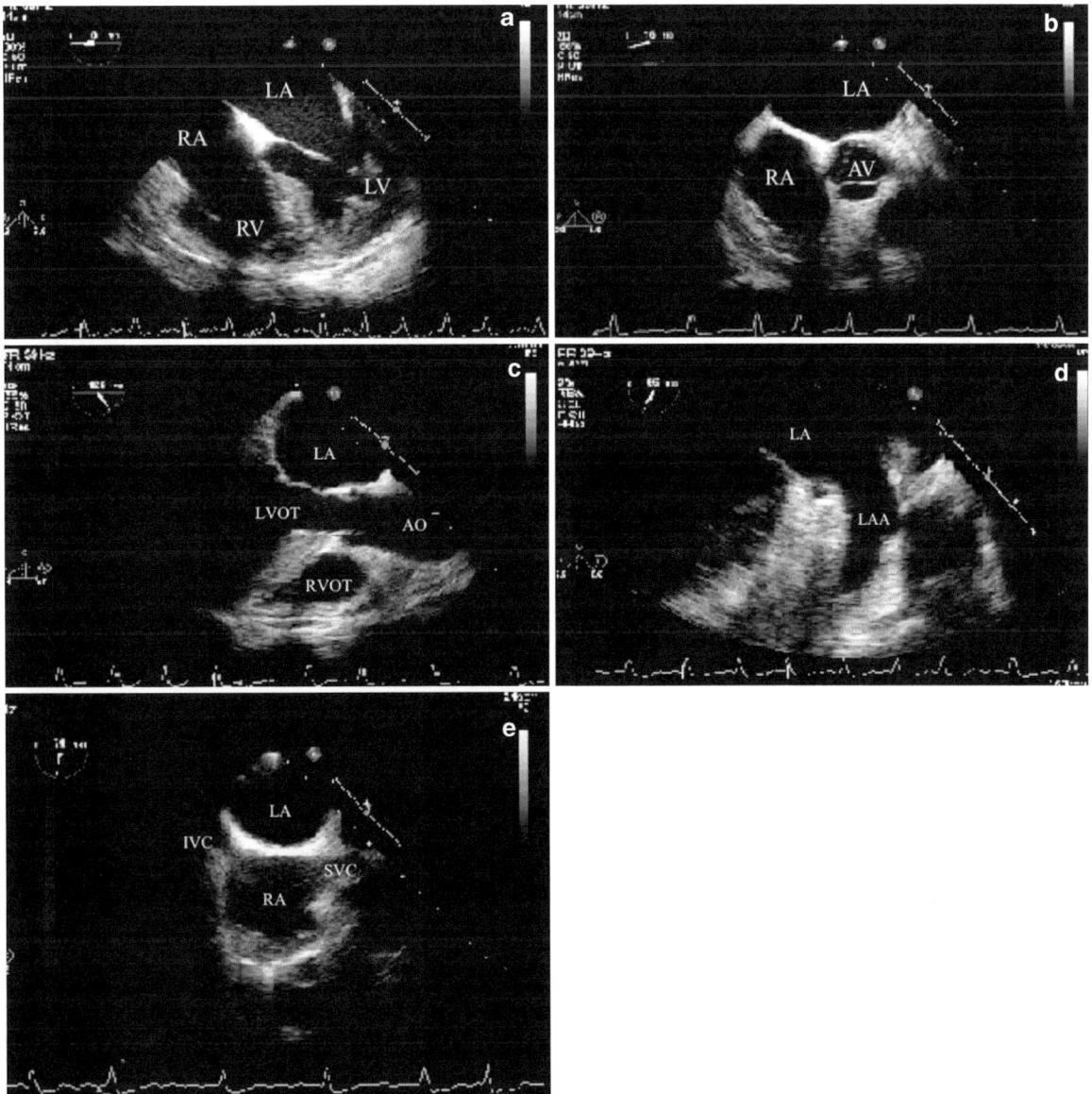

Fig. 3.4 TEE views: (**a**) Four-chamber view (0°) clearly displays left and right atria and ventricle, two atrioventricular valves, and atrial septum. (**b**) Short-axis view of aorta (16°) shows atrial septum, aorta, tricuspid valve, and right ventricular outflow tract, and therefore is useful to assess relationship between ASD and aorta. (**c**) Long-axis view of left ventricle and aorta (nearly 120°) shows the left ventricular outflow tract, aortic valve, and ascending aorta, and therefore is useful to visualize VSD and aortic valve. (**d**) TEE at 60° shows the structure of the left atrial appendage. (**e**) Double-atrium view (90°) shows entire atrial septum, which is useful during ASD closure

vention of congenital heart disease and its strict indication requirements. Only echocardiography can correctly estimate the size of a congenital heart abnormality, relationship with surrounding structures, and other details needed to inform clinical decision making. Preoperative evaluation of patients' cardiac function, pulmonary artery pressure and other related information can predict the risk and prognosis of the operation. The information cannot be completely and correctly obtained only by angiography. By cooperating with each other, the guidance and monitoring of TTE for interventional therapy can minimize the dose of radiation and avoid radiation damage. Reported interventional procedure-related complications include pericardial effusion and aortic valve perforation caused by occluder and atrial rupture, etc. Although their incidence is low, their clinical consequences are serious. Therefore, appropriate follow-up is needed.

3.2 Use of Echocardiography in Percutaneous Interventional Therapy for Atrial Septal Defect

3.2.1 Pre-procedural Echocardiographic Diagnosis of ASD

Indications of percutaneous interventional therapy: In patients with isolated secundum ASD causing impaired functional capacity, right atrial and/or RV enlargement, and net left-to-right shunt sufficiently large to cause physiological sequelae (e.g., pulmonary–systemic blood flow ratio [Qp:Qs] ≥1.5:1) without cyanosis at rest or during exercise, transcatheter or surgical closure to reduce RV volume and improve exercise tolerance is recommended, provided that systolic PA pressure is less than 50% of systolic systemic pressure and pulmonary vascular resistance is less than one-third of the systemic vascular resistance. Accurate sizing of

the ASD is mandatory for subsequent optimal selection of the device. Which can be seen and measure the distance from the surrounding rim of the defect to superior and inferior vena cava in subcostal double-atrium view. The left-to-right atrial shunt should be estimated by color Doppler flow images (CDFI) in related views. The entrances of pulmonary veins into left atrium should be examined in multiple views to exclude total anomalous pulmonary venous connection.

Inclusion criteria for case selection of atrial defect differ in age and weight, while requirements on defect structure are consistent with traditional fluoroscopy-guided occlusion. Ultrasound enrollment criteria were: central atrial septal defect with defect diameter ≥5 mm, with increased right heart volume load; distance from the margin of the defect to the coronary sinus, upper and inferior vena cava and pulmonary vein ≥5 mm, to atrioventricular valve ≥7 mm.

Exclusion criteria are: Ostium primum and sinus venosus ASD; endocarditis; hemorrhagic diseases; thrombosis was present at the occlusion site and the catheter insertion site; right to left shunting secondary to severe pulmonary hypertension, severe myocarditis or valve diseases unrelated to ASD; left atrium or left atrial appendage thrombosis; and partial or total anomalous pulmonary venous connection.

3.2.2 Echocardiography for Monitoring ASD Closure

Atrial septal defect (ASD) closure is now routinely performed using a percutaneous approach under echocardiographic guidance especially TTE.

Methods of TTE guidance: The position and size of ASD are evaluated in parasternal views, and indications are reconfirmed (Fig. 3.5) before puncture. Probe is placed in subcostal position to show IVC and monitor catheter advancement through IVC to the right atrium (Fig. 3.6a).

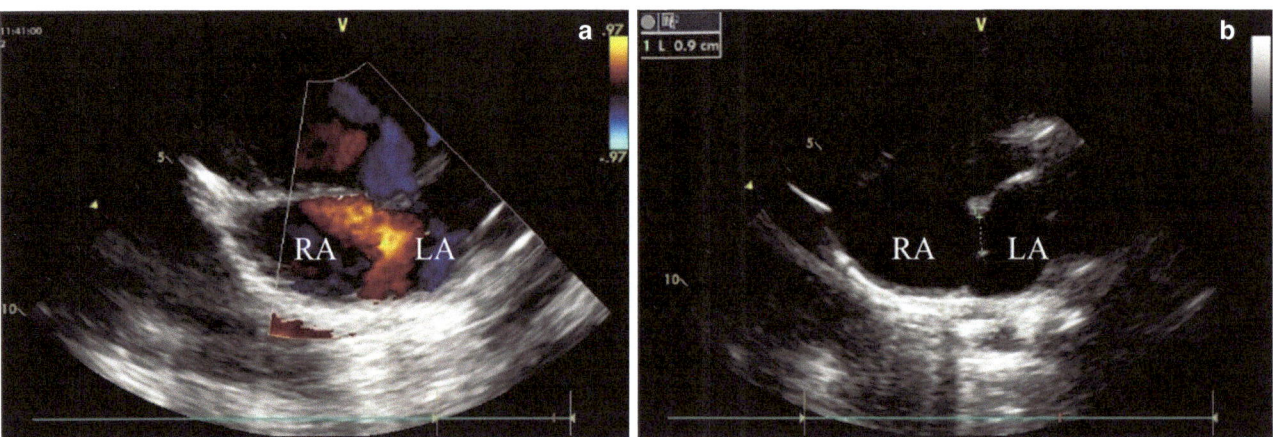

Fig. 3.5 TTE scanning for ASD: (**a**) The parasternal four-chamber view with color Doppler shows the left-to-right atrial shunt. (**b**) The diameter of the ASD is 9 mm

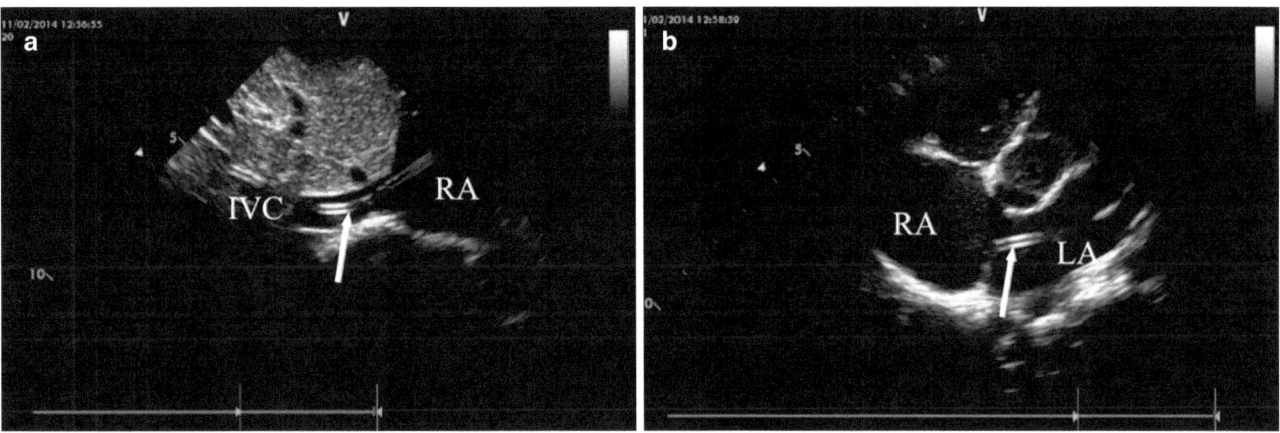

Fig. 3.6 TTE scanning for catheter: (**a**) Subcostal view shows that the catheter (↑) is in inferior vena cava. (**b**) The parasternal four-chamber view shows that the catheter (↑) is in the left atrium from the right atrium through the ASD

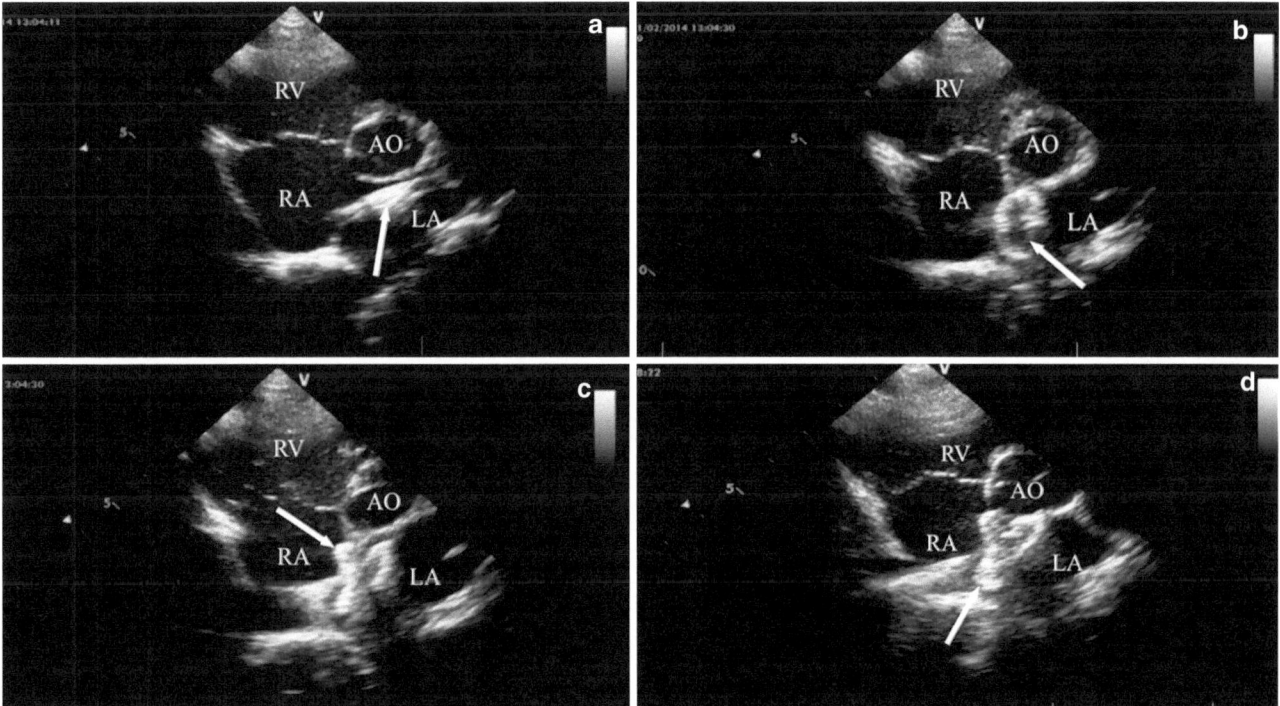

Fig. 3.7 TTE scanning for occluder: (**a**) Parasternal short-axis view shows that the catheter (↑) was into left atrium from right atrium through ASD; (**b**) The same view shows that the left atrial side of the occluder (↑) was deployed, and the position is normal. (**c**) The right atrial side of the occluder (↑) was completely deployed, the position and shape of the occluder are normal. (**d**) The parasternal short-axis view at aorta level shows that the occluder (↑) is completely released, and the relationship between the occluder and the surrounding structure was normal

Catheter position is then visualized in parasternal four-chamber view, and it is guided across the ASD (Fig. 3.6b) as is the delivery sheath. Under the short-axis view at the aorta level, the delivery sheath is detected, you should monitor it through the ASD (Fig. 3.7a). The occluder is placed in delivery sheath and into the right atrium and then to release it at the left atrial portion (Fig. 3.7b). Pull the left atrium umbrella back to the atrial septum and to release the right atrium part. Multiple views are used to assess occluder position, release sufficiency, the distance from bicuspid valve and tricuspid valve, valve function, and occluder edge clamping without fracture (Fig. 3.7d). Make sure no residual shunt flow by color Doppler (Fig. 3.8a). Coronary sinus and pulmonary venous flow should be carefully examined. After excluding the above problems, the occluder is released under guidance of apical four-chamber view (Fig. 3.8b). Finally, the position, shape, and surrounding structure of the occluder were observed again to determine whether it is successful.

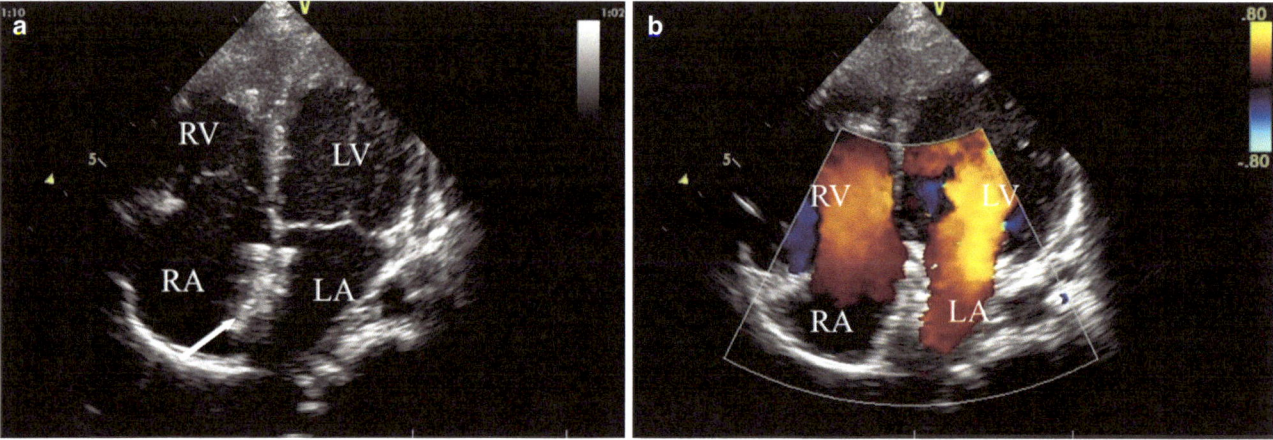

Fig. 3.8 Apical four-chamber view shows: (**a**) the position of ASD occluder (↑); (**b**) the color Doppler imaging indicates that there was no residual atrial septal shunt between left and right atrium, and the mitral and tricuspid valvular function was normal without regurgitation

However, TTE is limited by the conditions of the acoustic window, and it is impossible to clearly show the structure of the heart cavity in some cases, including obesity, barrel chest, and sternal deformity. In addition, TTE image quality and display range are not as good as TEE. For patients with difficult ASD, such as ASD margin is not ideal, large ASD, or ASD is closer to the superior and inferior vena cava, it is safer to be guided by TEE.

The content need to observe and monitor with TEE is consistent with TTE. The sonographer needs to flexibly use the transesophageal ultrasound to display the structure of the atrium. The common views include: the distance between defect and mitral or tricuspid valves pre-procedure at 0°; whether there is a touch between defect and mitral or tricuspid valves post-procedure; short-axis views at 45–60° show the edge of aorta and its contralateral side; the occluder is examined to determine if it is "encircled" rather than squeezed by the aorta; the pre-procedural distances between defect and superior and inferior vena cava are examined in double-atrial view at 120° to determine if the occluder is in close contact with vena cava openings. Overall, TEE views should be flexibly used to assess relationships among ASD, occluder, and intra-atrial structure.

3.2.3 Follow-Up Using Echocardiography After ASD Closure

- After closure, echocardiographic follow-up should be performed mainly to evaluate.
- Positioning and shape of occluder: In parasternal short-axis view at the aortic valve level and parasternal four-chamber view, left and right atria are examined to determine if occluder fits the ASD closely and firmly without displacement or dislodgment. Color Doppler flow image can show that is there any interatrial shunt.

- Pericardial cavity status: presence and volume of pericardial effusion.
- Recovery of right atrial and ventricular diameter.

3.3 Use of Echocardiography in Percutaneous Balloon Pulmonary Valvuloplasty for Pulmonary Stenosis

3.3.1 Pre-procedural Diagnosis of Pulmonary Stenosis

- The pulmonary valve activity curve is shown to be deepened (>4 mm), with extended opening time and thickened right ventricular wall.
- In 2D echocardiography (Fig. 3.9):
  1. Parasternal long-axis view shows right ventricular outflow tract, right ventricular wall thickening and cavity size, pulmonary valve thickening, and limitation of pulmonary artery valve opening.
  2. The parasternal short axis at aorta level shows the aortic valve, right ventricular outflow tract, pulmonary valve, and pulmonary artery structure. This view shows thickening of the pulmonary valve and enhanced echo density; the opening of the valve is restricted which presented as a dome sign; the pulmonary valve annulus is normal or small, and the main pulmonary artery is dilated; the secondary change is right ventricular wall hypertrophy. A modified intercostal attempt to show the short axis of the pulmonary valve, manifested as a thickening of the pulmonary valve, showing that the number of valves is three-, two- or single-valve deformity, and can also indicate the presence of muscular hypertrophy and stenosis in the outflow tract.

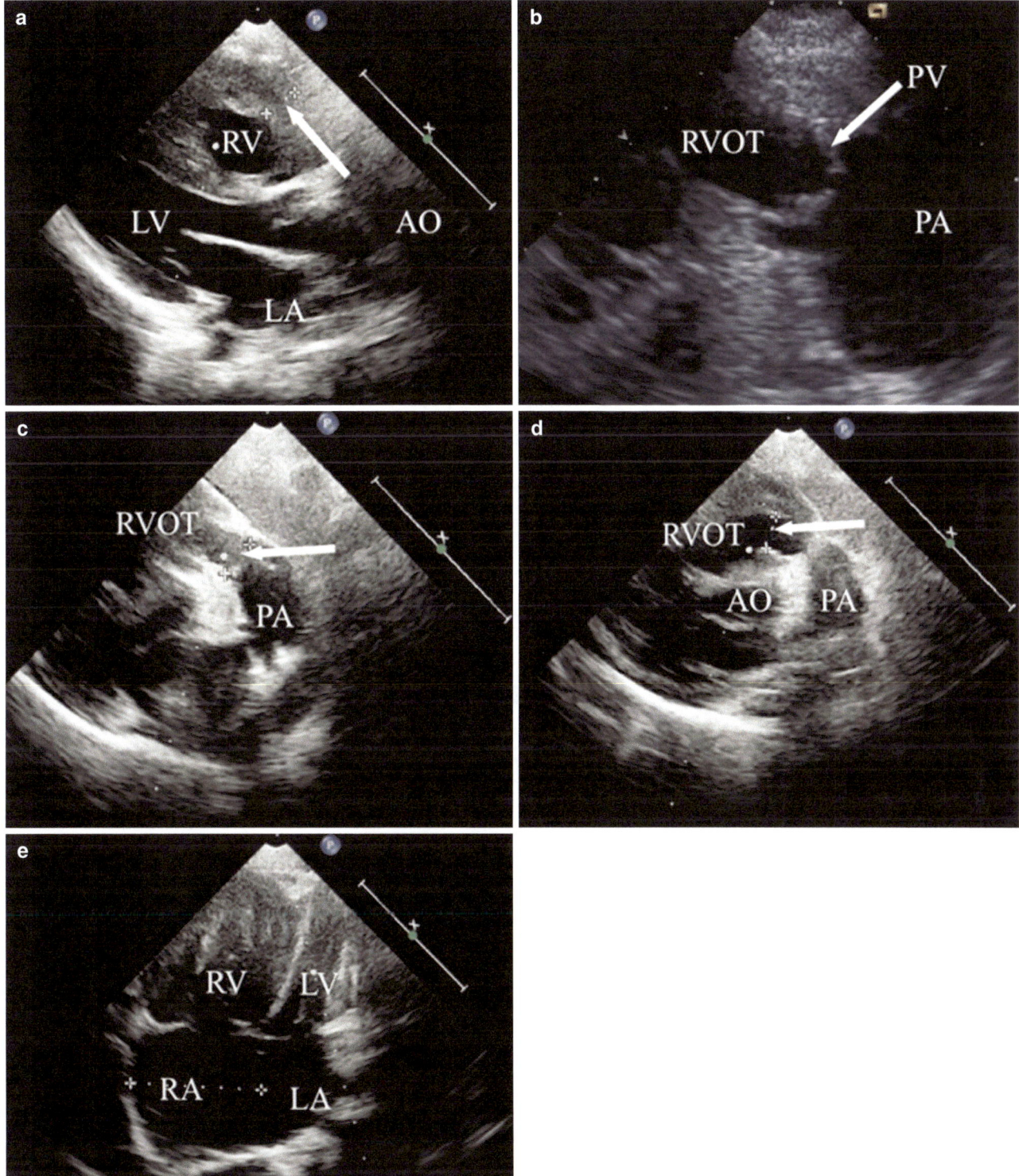

Fig. 3.9 2D left parasternal long-axis view shows a significantly thickened right ventricular wall (↑) (**a**), parasternal short-axis view shows thickened pulmonary valve (↑) (**b**), and allows measurement of pulmonary valve ring diameter (↑) (**c**), parasternal short-axis view of great arteries shows right ventricular outflow tract hypertrophy and measurement of its inner diameter (↑) (**d**), apical four-chamber view shows significantly enlarged right ventricle, a deviation in the left atrial septum, significantly thickened right ventricular wall, and slightly enlarged cavity (**e**)

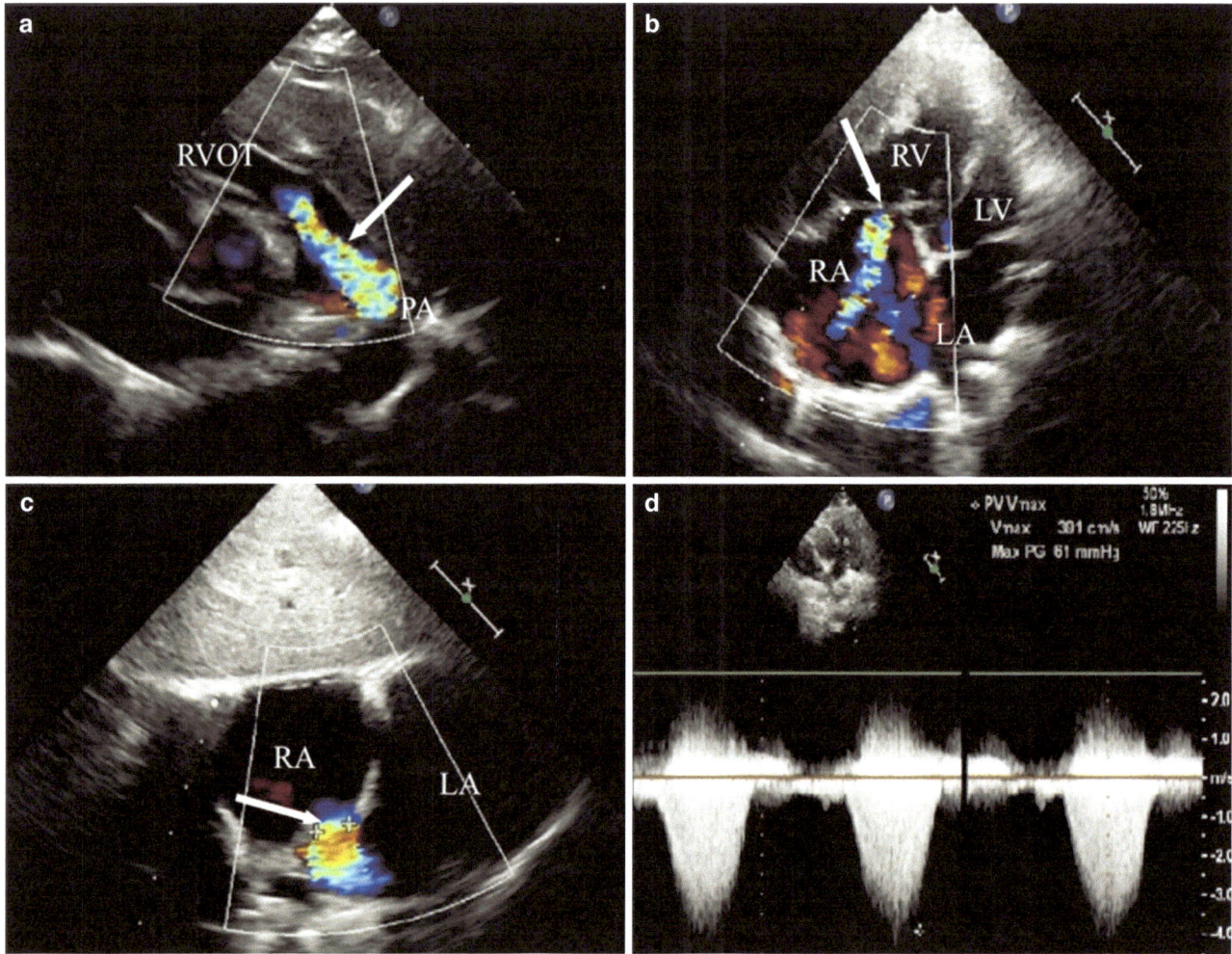

Fig. 3.10 Color Doppler shows the high velocity of pulmonary valve blood flow (↑) with aliasing (**a**); obvious tricuspid valve regurgitation (↑) (**b**); subcostal view shows patent foramen ovale with right-to-left atrial shunt (↑) (**c**); continuous wave Doppler shows high velocity of pulmonary valve blood flow (**d**)

3. Subcostal long-axis view can show right ventricular outflow tract, pulmonary valve, main pulmonary artery, left and right pulmonary arteries.
4. Apical four-chamber view shows enlargement of the right atrium and ventricle, thickening of the trabecular muscles, and reduction of the cardiac chamber.

- Doppler echocardiography (Fig. 3.10)
  1. Color Doppler shows high velocity of blood flow through the stenotic pulmonary valve orifice, with bright aliasing and turbulence in pulmonary artery.
  2. PW allows to measure the velocity of blood flow in right ventricular outflow tract, which should be a low-velocity, laminar flow spectrum under the pulmonary valve.
  3. CW allows measuring the high velocity of blood flow through pulmonary valve orifice, and calculating transvalvular gradient.

4. If the pressure gradient is ≥20 mmHg, the pulmonary artery stenosis is mild, and if ≥40 mmHg, treatment is needed. In patients with simple pulmonary stenosis, the higher the velocity of tricuspid regurgitation, the more severe the pulmonary stenosis.

3.3.2 Key Points of Echocardiographic Evaluation Before Pulmonary Stenosis Valvuloplasty

Echocardiography screening usually is performed for patients >3 years old.

The indication of balloon valvuloplasty for pulmonary artery stenosis is patients with simple pulmonary stenosis, pressure gradient ≥40 mmHg.

The contraindications are: pulmonary inferior funnel stenosis; double-chambered right ventricle; pulmonary stenosis associated with congenital subvalvular or superior valvular stenosis; and pulmonary stenosis with severe pulmonary valvular dysplasia. The congenital heart diseases should be treated by surgery.

3.3.3 Echocardiographic Guidance and Monitoring During Pulmonary Valvuloplasty

The benefits of echocardiography monitor during pulmonary valvuloplasty procedure are: (1) to guide operator to place the balloon in the right position and improves success rate of valvuloplasty; (2) relieves right ventricular outflow tract obstruction due to infundibular muscle spasm, and reduces complication rate.

3.3.3.1 Pulmonary Valvuloplasty Guided and Monitored by TEE

Place the TEE probe in the mid esophagus at about 40° view to show the right ventricular outflow tract and pulmonary valve, one should place the ring of the balloon catheter in the center of pulmonary artery orifice. Under TEE monitoring, the balloon is inflated to expand the pulmonary valve; a suitable size of balloon should be selected according to the size of pulmonary annulus. After balloon dilatation, heart rate

and blood pressure should be monitored; the velocity of blood flow through pulmonary artery valve should be measured. Operators should observe that is there any pulmonary valve or tricuspid valve regurgitation; and record the velocity of tricuspid valve regurgitation (Fig. 3.11). Interventions must pay attention to pericardial effusions and may develop right ventricular outflow tract muscle spasms due to catheter insertion stimulation. The procedure is considered successful if pressure gradient through pulmonary valve is <36 mmHg (Figs. 3.11 and 3.12).

3.3.3.2 Pulmonary Valvuloplasty Guided by TTE

As balloon catheter get in IVC, operator can send the balloon catheter through right atrium, tricuspid valve, right ventricular outflow tract, pulmonary valve orifice to pulmonary artery under TTE guidance. The parasternal short-axis view at great arteries level is routinely used to monitor the pulmonary valvuloplasty procedure.

3.3.4 Echocardiographic Follow-Up After Pulmonary Valvuloplasty Procedure

The follow-up echocardiography examination should be scheduled at 24 h, 3 days, and 1, 3, 6 and 12 months post-procedure.

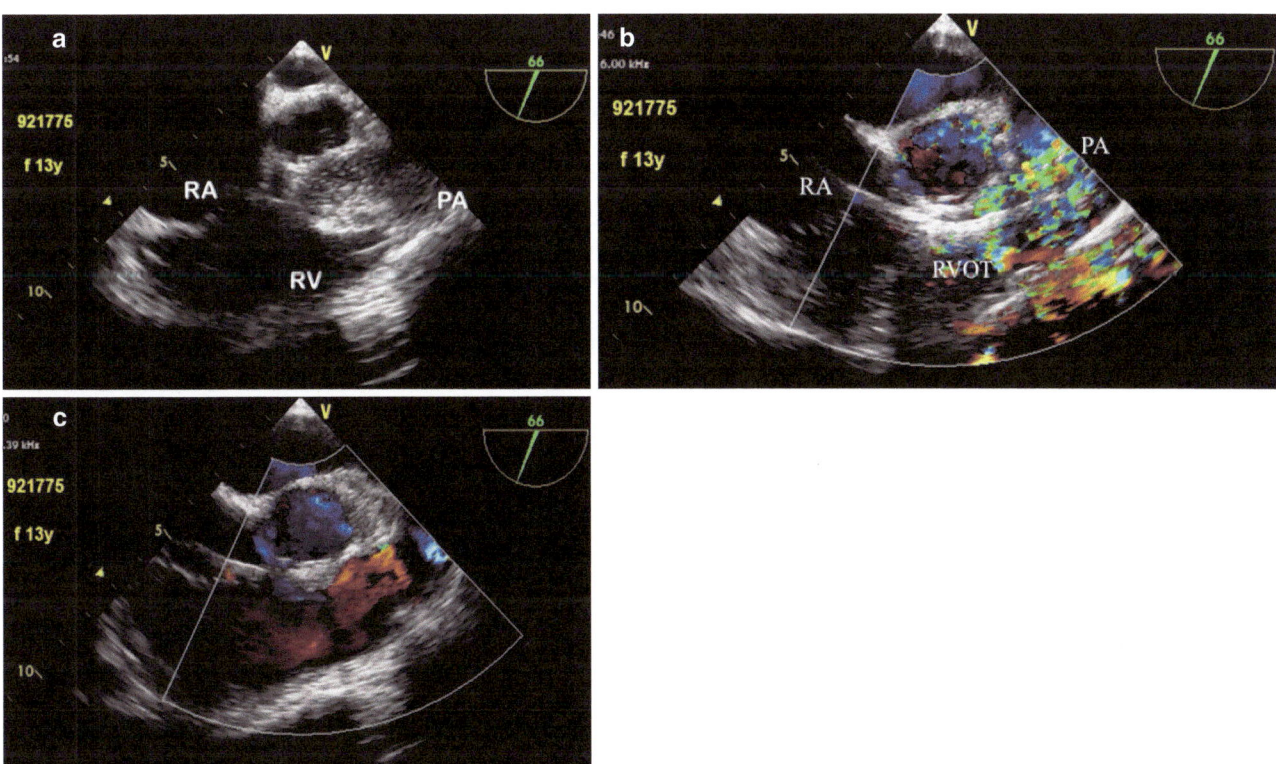

Fig. 3.11 TEE probe in mid of esophagus at 66° shows the dilated balloon in the center of the pulmonary valve orifice (**a**); increased blood flow after first dilatation (**b**); significantly increased blood flow at the pulmonary artery valve after another dilatation (**c**)

Fig. 3.12 Continuous wave Doppler recording from parasternal short-axis view: The peak velocity of pulmonary valve is 161 cm/s

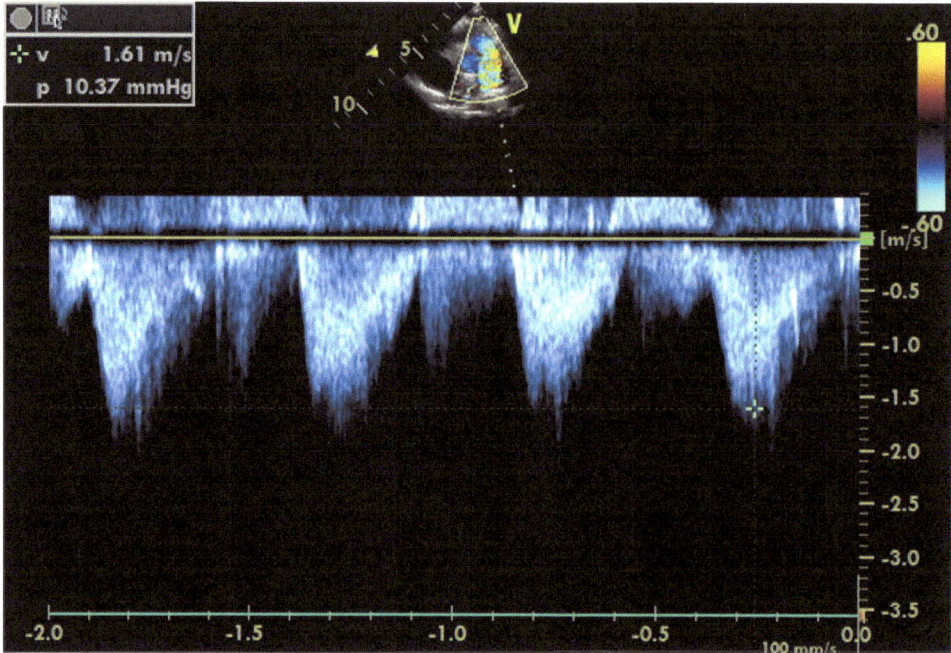

The examination focuses on pressure gradient across pulmonary valve, tricuspid regurgitation, right heart size and cardiac function.

3.4   Use of Echocardiography in Percutaneous Interventions for Patent Ductus Arteriosus (PDA)

3.4.1   Pre-procedural Echocardiographic Diagnosis of PDA

In cases with patent ductus arteriosus, echocardiography examination will show left heart volume overload, i.e., left atrial and ventricular dilation. In parasternal short-axis view at aortic valve level or suprasternal view, there is an abnormal canal between the main pulmonary artery and descending aorta with high velocity of blood flow by color Doppler image (CDFI), which is continuous retrograde blood flow during cardiac cycle.

The pre-procedural evaluation for interventional closure of PDA includes the assessment of:

- The diameter of the aortic side and the pulmonary artery side of the PDA and the length of the PDA; in addition, whether the aorta or pulmonary artery can be displayed on the same view should also be noted.
- If patients with left-to-right and more rarely right-to-left shunt through PDA indicate that the patient is associated with pulmonary artery hypertension.

- Degree of atrioventricular valve regurgitation and other heart diseases should be carefully examined.

3.4.2   Echocardiographic Guidance During PDA Closure Procedure

The suprasternal or parasternal short-axis view at aortic level should be used to guide percutaneous PDA closure procedure. The guide wire is advanced to the pulmonary artery either antegrade via femoral vein through right atrium using parasternal short-axis view at aortic valve level to guide (Fig. 3.13) or retrograde via femoral artery through descending aorta and patent arterial duct using suprasternal view to guide (Fig. 3.14). The parasternal short-axis view at aortic valve level should be used to monitor the guide wire, sheath, and occluder delivery, which is sent to the descending aorta. The occluder surface should be closely fit in the PDA without excessively protruding into descending aorta, or left pulmonary artery. Operator should make sure there is no residual arterial shunting, and normal flow in both descending aorta and left pulmonary artery by color Doppler (Fig. 3.15). PDA closure is considered successful if the velocity of forward flow of descending aorta is <2 m/s and that of left pulmonary artery is <1.5 m/s. Otherwise, the occluder position should be adjusted. The above process should be confirmed repeatedly using the suprasternal and parasternal short-axis view at aortic valve level.

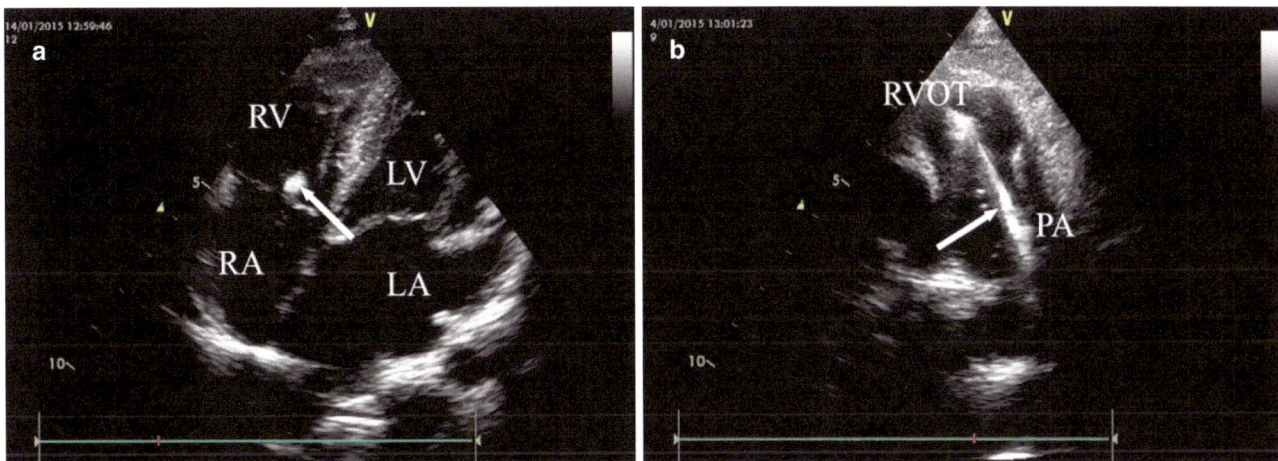

Fig. 3.13 PDA closure procedure is performed via femoral vein. The TTE apical four-chamber view shows that the guide wire (↑) is advanced through the right atrium, tricuspid valve into right ventricle (**a**). The parasternal short-axis view at aortic valve level shows that the guide wire (↑) is advanced through arterial duct into pulmonary artery (**b**)

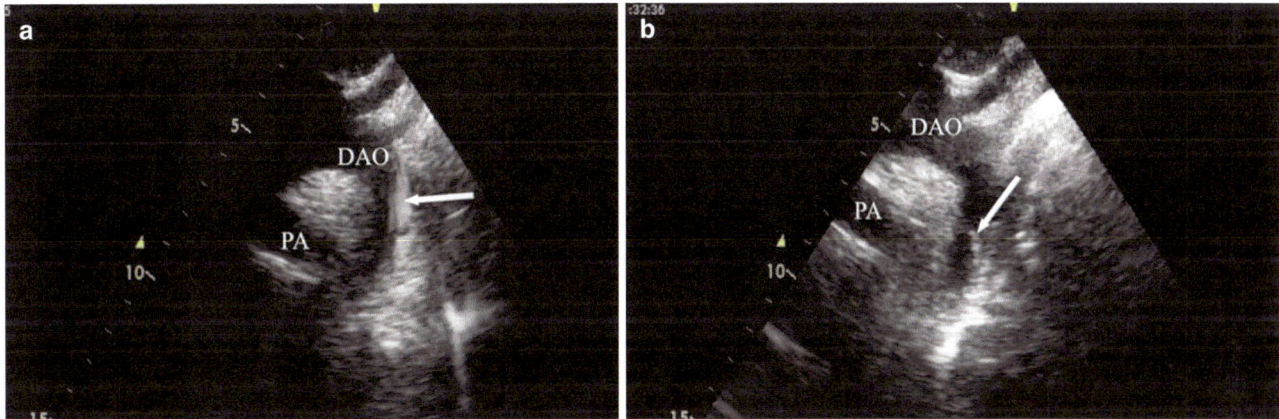

Fig. 3.14 PDA closure procedure is performed via femoral artery. TTE suprasternal view indicates the guide wire (↑) through the descending aorta (**a**) and arterial duct into the pulmonary artery (↑) (**b**)

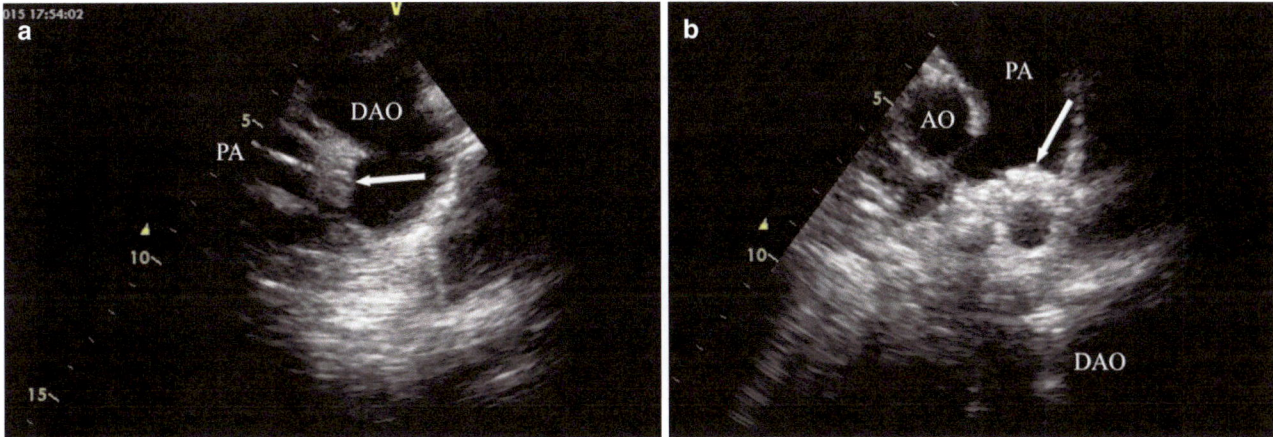

Fig. 3.15 Transcutaneous occlusion of the PDA: The TTE suprasternal view shows that the occluder (↑) had reached the position of PDA, the aortic side disc had been deployed (**a**), and the short axis of the aorta shows that the occluder of the pulmonary artery side (↑) was completely deployed, the waist is stuck in the PDA, the occluder disc surfaces on both sides are completely open, and the fit is tight (**b**)

3.4.3 Echocardiographic Follow-Up After PDA Closure

Echocardiographic follow-up should be performed early after PDA closure to evaluate:

- Echocardiography should be performed in patients soon after PDA closure and at 24 h, 3 days, and 1, 3, 6 and 12 months post-procedure, to evaluate the position of occluder and is there any significant ductal shunt during follow-up.
- The pericardial cavity: detect presence and amount of pericardial effusion.
- Descending aorta or left pulmonary artery stenosis: The inner diameter, velocity of blood flow, and other parameters in descending aorta and left pulmonary artery should be examined by 2D echocardiography and CDFI. If the velocity of forward flow in descending aorta is <2 m/s and that of left pulmonary artery is <1.5 m/s, the PDA closure procedure is considered successful.
- The parameter of cardiac chamber remodeling after PDA closure.

3.5 Use of Echocardiography in Percutaneous Closure of Ventricular Septal Defect

3.5.1 Pre-procedural Echocardiographic Diagnosis of VSD

- The technique for VSD closure starts with a detailed echocardiographic examination, typically using TEE, to carefully evaluate the size of the defect and its relationship with adjacent cardiac structures using multiple cardiac views.

- Examination
  1. TTE should be performed before the procedure. The size, relationship with tricuspid, pulmonary, and aortic valves, and supraventricular crest of VSD should be evaluated using different cardiac views to determine the classification of VSD.
  2. Ventricular shunts and their direction are evaluated with color Doppler image to measure shunt volume, pulmonary–systemic blood flow ratio [Qp:Qs].
  3. The velocity of shunt and tricuspid regurgitation should be measured by continuous wave Doppler to estimate right ventricle and pulmonary artery pressures.
  4. The sizes of cardiac cavities, right ventricular outflow tract and pulmonary artery, especially left ventricle should be measured to evaluate the left heart volume load status and function.
  5. The other cardiac congenital abnormality should be carefully scanned.
  6. Patients with elevated pulmonary artery pressure, aortic valve regurgitation associated with VSD, or a defect too large for the device were not candidates for transcatheter closure.

- Echocardiography evaluation of perimembranous VSD
  1. Parasternal left ventricular long-axis view shows left ventricular cavity enlargement.
  2. The aortic valve, right ventricular outflow tract, pulmonary valve, and pulmonary artery could be clearly seen in parasternal short-axis view at aortic valve level. The probe should be slightly moved downward to better visualize discontinuity in membranous ventricular septum. A high velocity of left-to-right shunt with colorful embedding could be seen during systole by color Doppler (Fig. 3.16). The velocity of left-to-right shunt through VSD and tricuspid valve regurgitation should be measured by alignment of echocardiography continuous

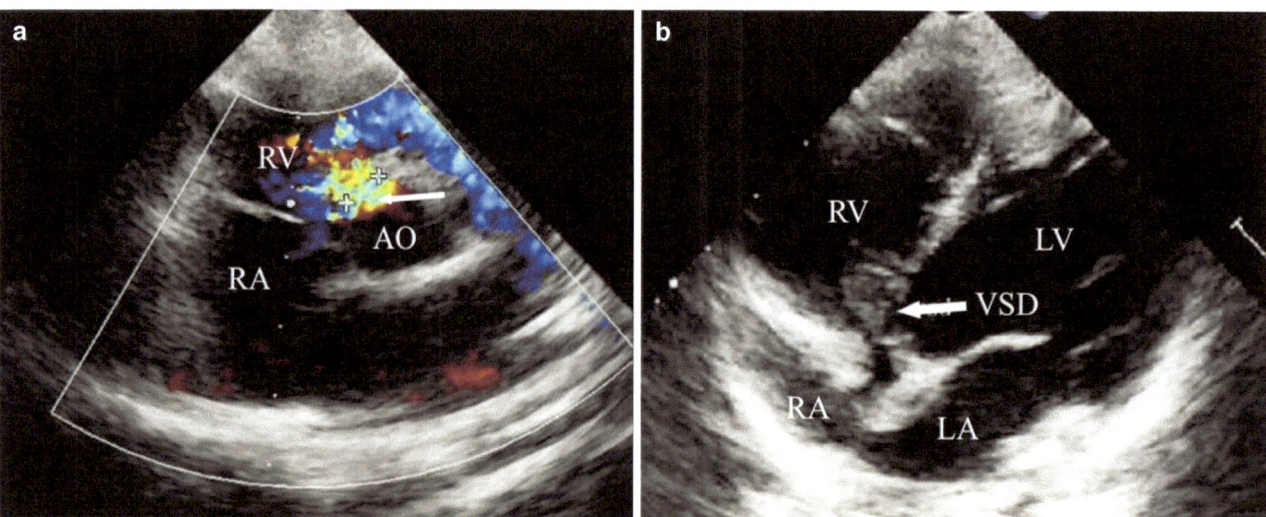

Fig. 3.16 Parasternal short-axis view with color Doppler image shows the perimembranous VSD (↑) (**a**); modified four-chamber view shows perimembranous VSD (↑) (**b**)

wave Doppler line parallel to shunt or regurgitation flow direction for estimating the gradient between left and right ventricular pressure and pulmonary artery pressure.

3. Ventricle septal defect measurement

The echo drop out nearby aortic right coronary valve at interventricular septum can be seen. The VSD size and the distance between VSD and aortic, tricuspid valves should be measured.

3.5.2 Key Points on Echocardiographic Evaluation Before Interventional VSD Closure

VSDs are classified into perimembranous, infundibular, and muscular types according to location.

Perimembranous VSD is the most common and the optimal indication for percutaneous intervention. Quantity, size and shape of defects, and the distance between VSD and aortic valve (shortest distance in left ventricular long axis or apical five-chamber view) should be measured. Some perimembranous defects protrude into the right ventricle as a pouch or adhere to a tricuspid valve leaflet. In patients with pouch, the defect size and shape of the pouch, and the relationship between the pouch and tricuspid valve, number, size and shape of the effective shunts of right ventricular side of the VSD should be measured or evaluated. Traditionally, the distance between defects and aortic valve should be >2 mm. However, using the application of eccentricity occluder, this condition can be appropriately relaxed to 2 mm.

Because infundibular VSD is near the aortic valve, attention should be paid to the possibility of occluder effects on aortic valve. Because the sub-arterial ventricular septal defect is close to the aortic valve, it is necessary to guard against the influence of the occluder on the aortic valve, especially the larger ventricular septal defect, and the defect is close to the aortic valve and pulmonary valve, so the effect of occluder on the valve is almost inevitable and it is not suitable for occlusion treatment under the current technical conditions.

The occluders used for patients with muscular VSD are different from patients with perimembranous VSD. In addition to the size and location of the defect, the right side of interventricular septum should be estimated by echocardiography. Since the placement of the occluder requires the catheter bevel to be too large, it is difficult to perform the closure procedure for a patient with a defect near the apex.

3.5.3 Echocardiographic Monitoring During VSD Closure

TEE and TTE have advantages and disadvantages that influence their selection for monitoring purposes according to anesthesia modality, intubation status, and acoustic window limitations. TEE avoids interference by thoracic cavity deformity and pulmonary air yielding a clearer monitoring image; however, the esophageal probe may be painful to fully conscious patients who might not tolerate it for a long time. In contrast, TTE is more convenient and painless for patients; however, acoustic windows may be suboptimal for some patients in the supine position. The patient should be selected according to whether there is a clear image of TTE.

At present, percutaneous interventional occlusion for ventricular septal defect is mainly through the femoral artery and trans-jugular vein. Monitored and guided by echocardiography, the catheter route of the former is from ascending aorta to aortic valve to left ventricular outflow tract and to right ventricle. Therefore, the VSD occluder is first released on the right ventricular side: the route of the latter is from superior vena cava to right atrium to tricuspid valve to right ventricle through VSD to left ventricle. Therefore, the VSD occluder is first released on the left ventricular side.

- A clear ultrasound image is obtained and defect position is determined.
- Catheter and guide wire are localized in real time to direct guide wire advancement and position of the guide wire's proximal end. If the echocardiography image is not optimal for superior vena cava to right atrium, the probe angle should be carefully adjusted by rotation to provide accurate information to operators (Fig. 3.17).
- The effects of the catheter and guide wire on the heart structure should be monitored in real time to avoid damage to the aorta and tricuspid valves. In addition, multiple views should be used to monitor the effect on the surrounding structures when the occluder is released to avoid damage to the valve and aortic sinus.
- The operator should make sure that the defect occluder has been placed in the right place and fit the surrounding tissue tightly without residue shunt (Figs. 3.18 and 3.19) before and after occluder release
- Pericardium should be examined to observe that is there any pericardial effusion.

3.5.4 Echocardiography for Follow-Up of Ventricular Septal Defect Occlusion and Complications

Based on its precision, noninvasiveness, convenience, and low cost, TTE plays an important role in follow-up after VSD percutaneous closure. In addition to routine assessment of ventricular size, residual shunt, position and shape of occluder, and pericardial effusion, attention should be paid to the possible effects of occluder on the valves, secondary aortic or tricuspid regurgitation.

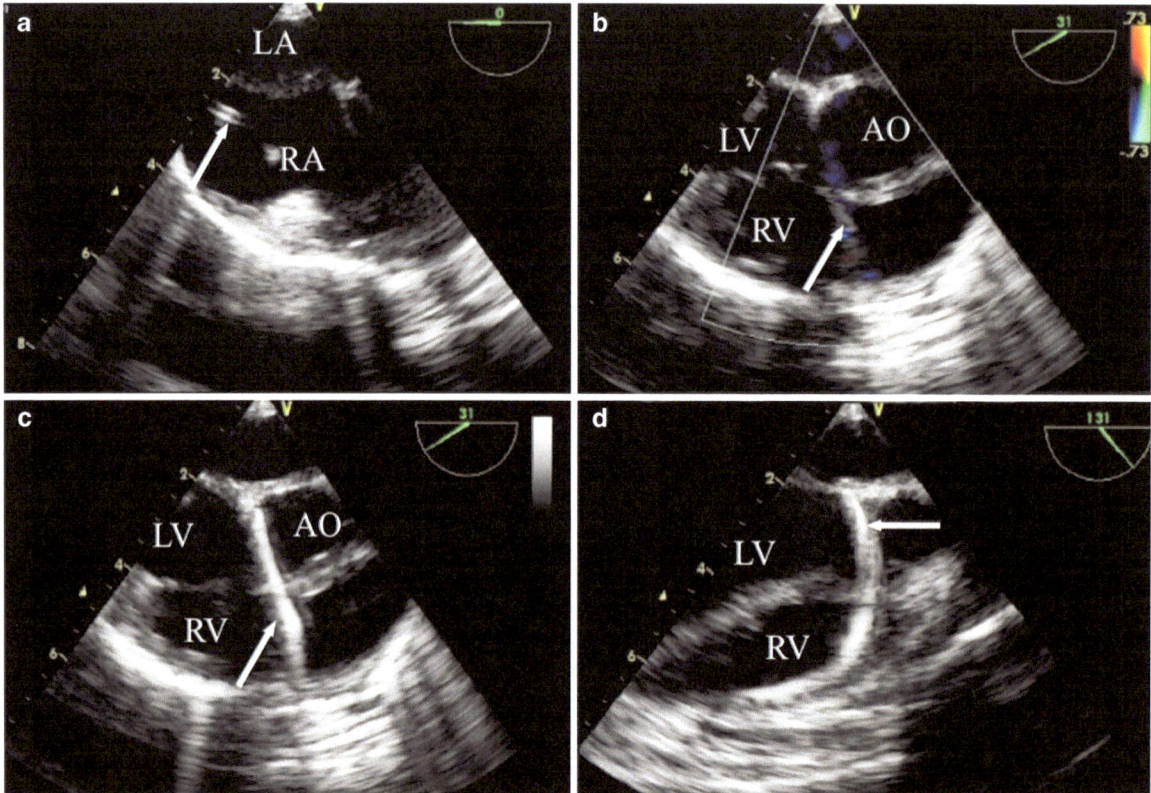

Fig. 3.17 TEE-guided VSD closure via jugular vein. The echo probe was in mid of esophagus at 0°, catheter (↑) is seen in the right atrium (**a**); The echo probe was in mid esophagus at 31°, guide wire (↑) is further advanced into the right ventricle through the tricuspid valve (**b**); guide wire (↑) has crossed VSD and entered left ventricular outflow tract (**c**), which also can be seen at 130° in left ventricle (↑) long-axis view (**d**)

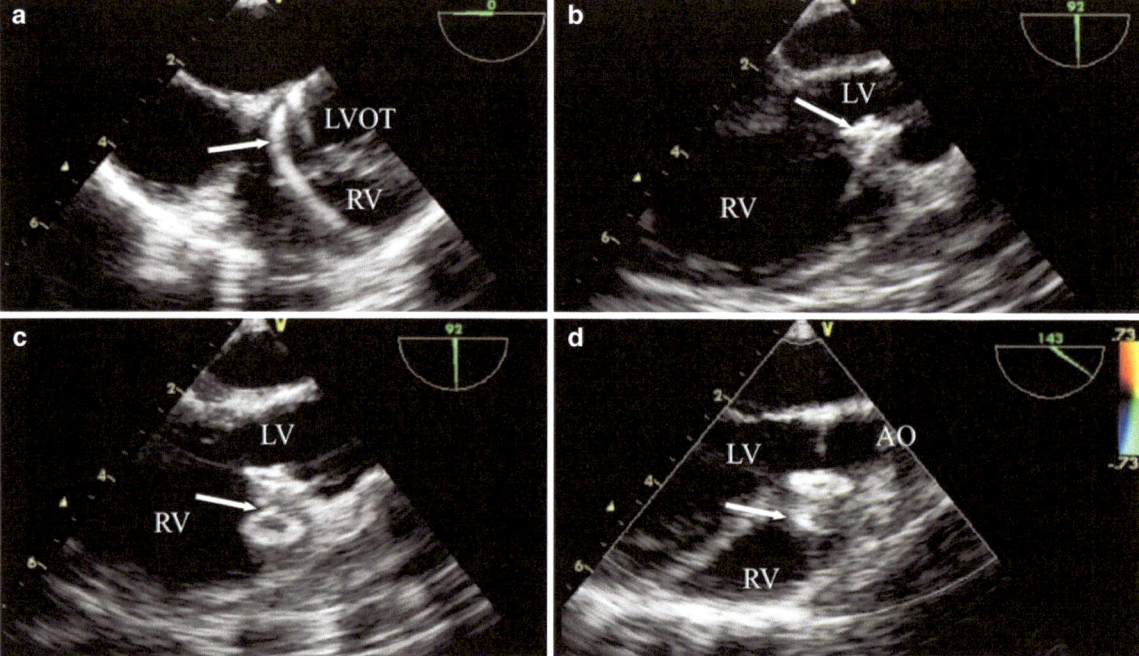

Fig. 3.18 TEE-guided VSD closure by femoral vein approach. The probe was in mid esophagus at 0°, the four-chamber view confirmed that guide wire (↑) has crossed the defect and entered the left ventricular outflow tract (**a**); at 90°, the parasternal short-axis view showed that the occluder (↑) of left ventricular side has been released (**b**), while the right ventricular side (↑) remains open (**c**); at about 140°, both of left and right ventricular sides of occluder (↑) have been released completely (**d**)

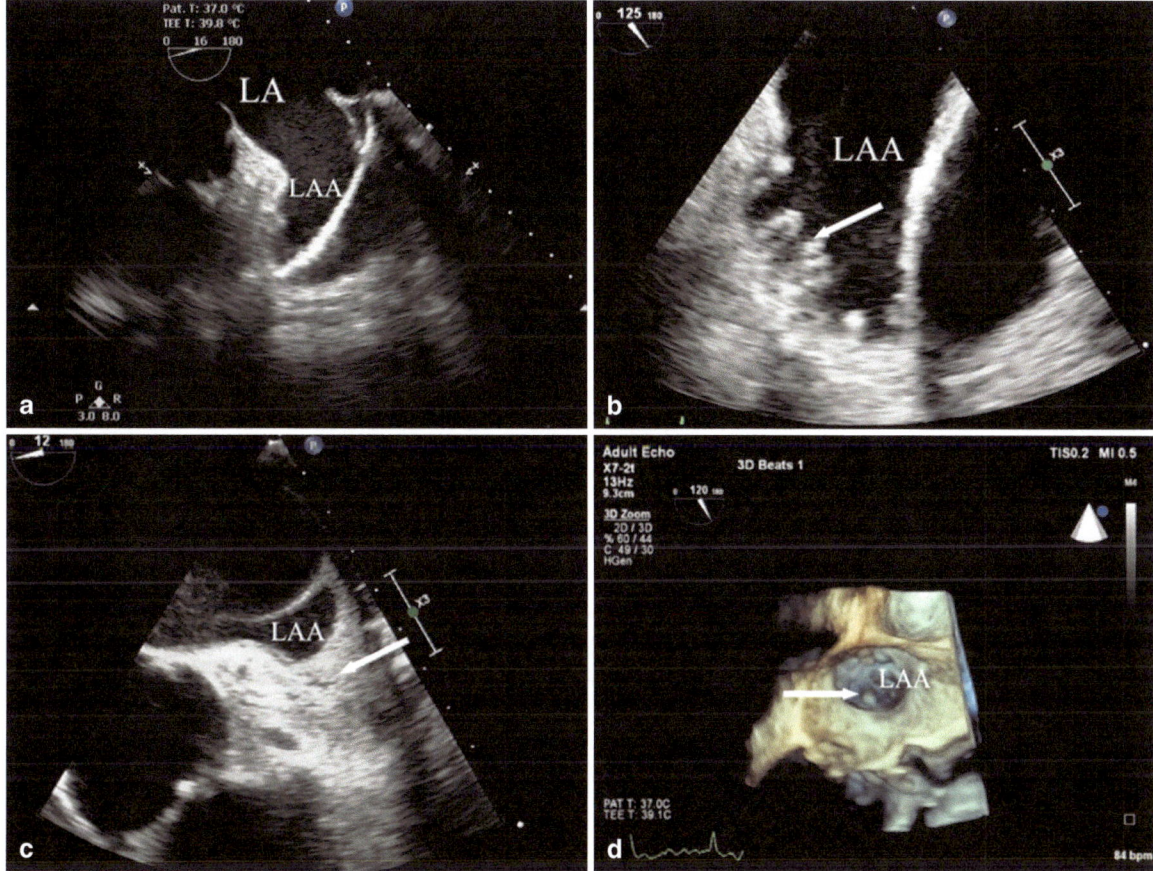

Fig. 3.19 Pre-procedural TEE screening for left atrial appendage occlusion. (**a**) Normal shape of left atrial appendage without thrombus; (**b**) Comb muscle (↑) in left atrial appendage without thrombus; (**c**) Thrombosis (↑) filling in left atrial appendage; (**d**) 3D-TEE shows thrombus in left atrial appendage (↑)

3.6   Use of Echocardiography in Left Atrial Appendage Occlusion

3.6.1   Pre-procedural Echocardiographic Diagnosis and Cases Screen

Pre-procedural TEE should be used to exclude left atrial appendage thrombus, to assess the shape of the left atrial appendage, measure the parameters of the left atrial appendage, to determine whether it is feasible to place the occluder in the left atrial appendage, and select the appropriate occluder (see Fig. 3.19).

Left atrial appendage measurements: The diameter of the orifice of the left atrial appendage, the maximum length of the main lobe of the left atrial appendage, and the depth of the left atrial appendage were measured at 0°, 45°, 90°, and 135°, respectively (see Fig. 3.20). (Different occluder products require different measurement.)

The choice of occluder: according to parameters of the left atrial appendage measured by TEE, the diameter of the occluder should be 20–40% larger than the diameters of the left atrial appendage.

3.6.2   Echocardiography for Monitoring Left Atrial Appendage Occlusion

The left atrial appendage can be fully displayed and evaluated by complete 0–180° multiplane of TEE. TEE is mainly used for guiding the transporting, placing occluder and evaluating immediately after percutaneous intervention. The percutaneous path of monitoring is: inferior vena cava-right atrium-atrial septum puncture-left atrium-left atrial appendage. The location of the atrial septum puncture is the key to the successful placement of the occluder. After successful septal puncture, delivery and placement of the occluder; firstly display and determine the position of the sheath in the left atrial appendage, and then to deliver the occluder into the left atrial appendage, and place the occluder in the left atrial appendage under TEE guidance. Then evaluate the positional relationship between the occluder and the left atrial appendage wall: during the placement of the occluder, the operator should observe the relationship and orientation of the occluder with the left atrial appendage and the left atrial wall and ensure that the main axis of the occluder and the long axis of the left atrial appendage are in one direction, and the position of the

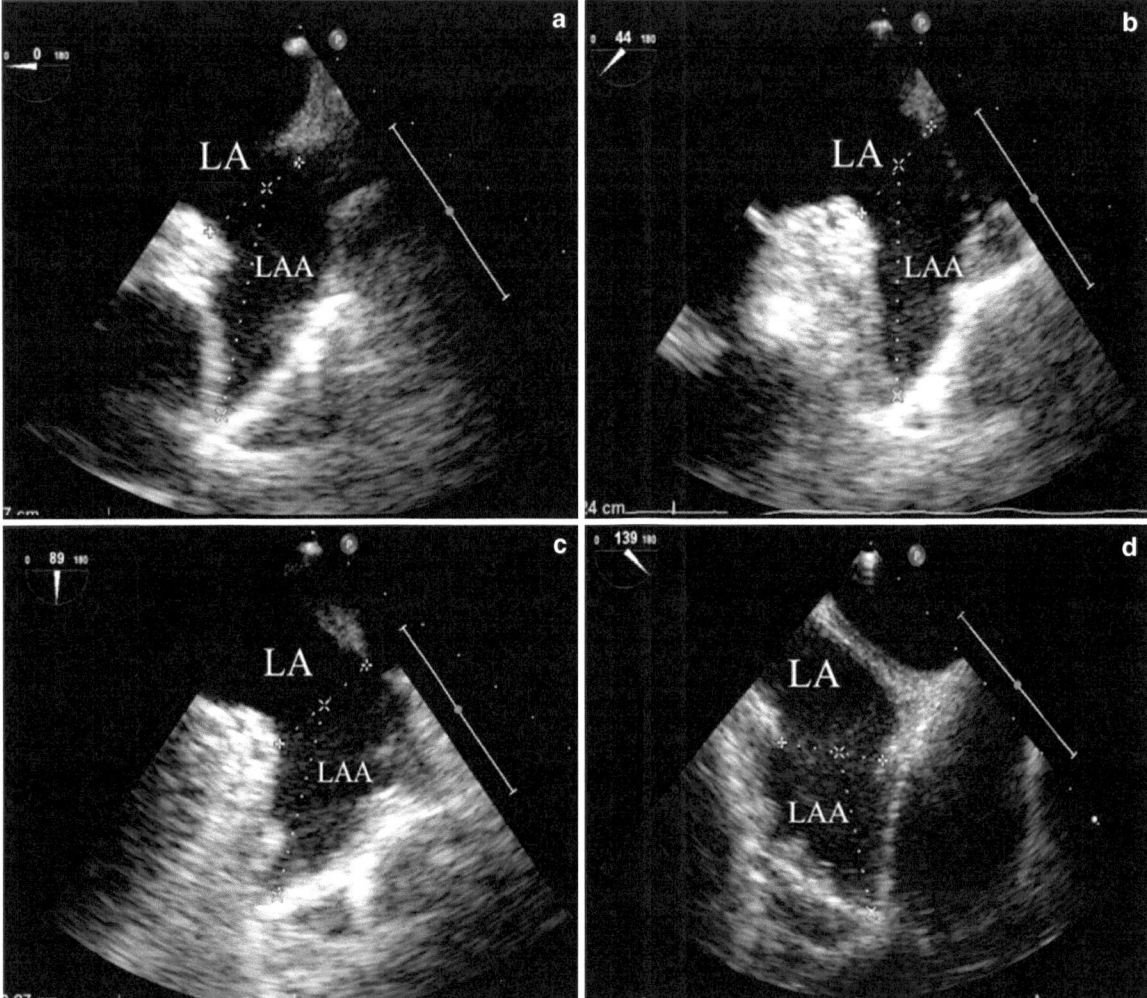

Fig. 3.20 TEE images shows the measurements of left atrial appendage at 0° (**a**), 44° (**b**), 89° (**c**), and 139° (**d**), respectively

occluder is accurate and stable. After placing the occluder in the LAA, whether there is any peri-occluder leakage and whether the occluder has adverse effects on the surrounding structures (such as the left superior pulmonary vein and the mitral valve) should be evaluated by TEE and then releases the occluder (see Figs. 3.21 and 3.22). After release, the position and shape of the occluder, the presence or absence of peri-occluder leakage, and adverse effects on the surrounding structure were evaluated again. The pericardial effusion should be monitored throughout the process.

3.6.3 Echocardiography for Follow-Up of Left Atrial Appendage Occlusion

After left atrial appendage occlusion, echocardiography examination should be performed before discharge and at 1, 6 months and 1 year after closure. If TTE images are not satisfied, TEE should be recommended.

1. The main contents of observation: The position, shape and the stability of the occluder, whether there is occluder displacement, or whether it affects the surrounding structure. Observe whether the surface of the occluder is smooth, and whether there is thrombus formation on or around the occluder.
2. Whether there is peri-occluder leakage. See Table 3.1.
3. Pericardial cavity: Is there any pericardial effusion.

3.7 Use of Echocardiography in Percutaneous Mitral Valve Stenosis Valvuloplasty

3.7.1 Echo Assessment of Mitral Stenosis

• M-mode echocardiography
  – Using M-mode in mitral stenosis to assess:
    1. Is the echo density of the anterior and posterior mitral leaflets enhanced?

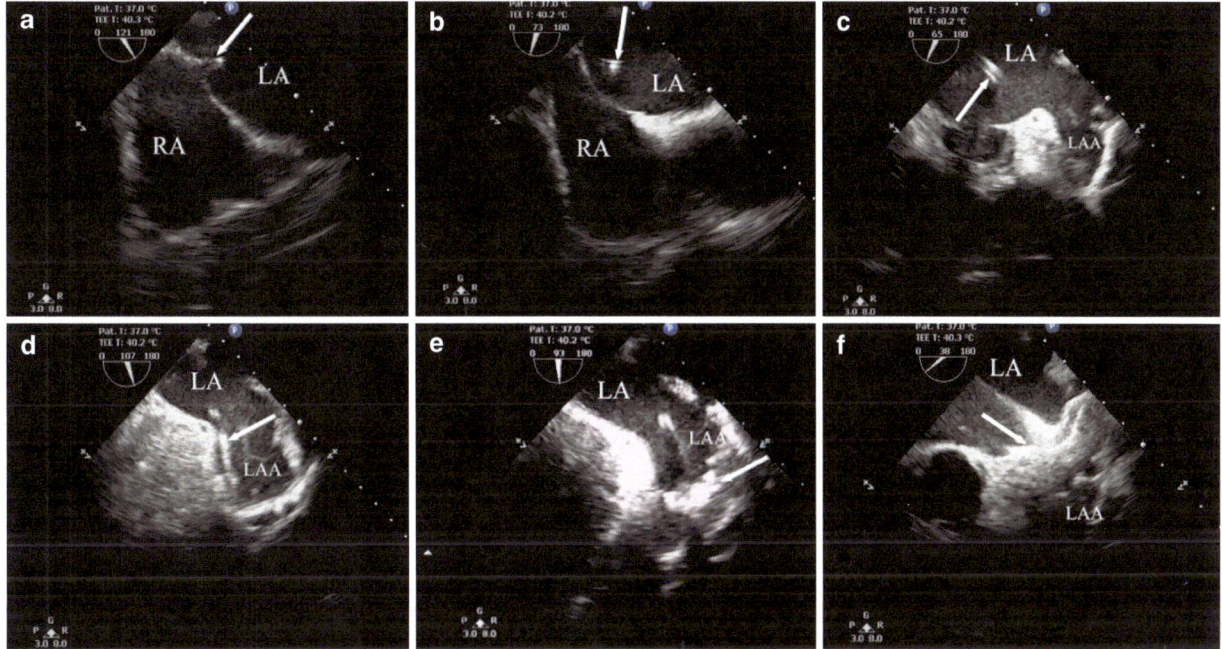

Fig. 3.21 Left atrial appendage occlusion monitoring by TEE. (**a**) Puncture the atrial septum (↑); (**b**) sheath (↑) was through atrial septal into the left atrium; (**c**) sheath (↑) was approach to left atrial appendage. (**d**) sheath (↑) enters the left atrial appendage; (**e**) occluder (↑) is delivered to the left atrial appendage; (**f**) determine the optimal location of occluder (↑) after release

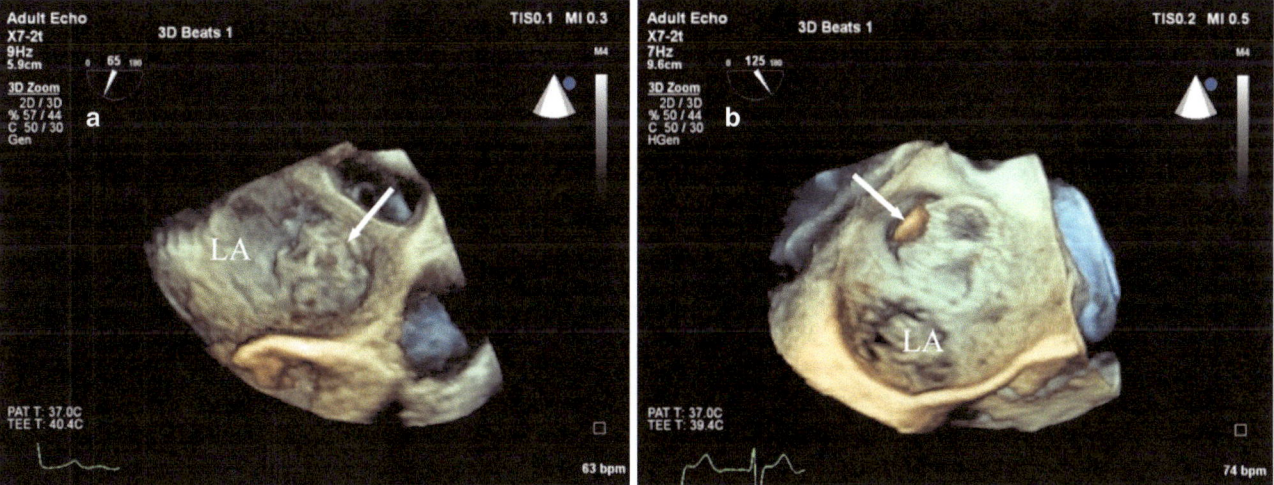

Fig. 3.22 3D-TEE image shows: (**a**) occluder (↑) was in good location and shape. (**b**) there was a trace of peri-occluder leakage (↑)

Table 3.1 Indicators of peri-occluder regurgitation severity evaluated by TEE color Doppler during procedure and follow-up

Color Doppler	Minor	Mild	Moderate	Severe
Peri-leakage width (mm)	<1	1–3	>3	Multiple color flows

2. Is there reduced excursion of the mitral leaflets during diastole?
3. Is there evidence of commissural fusion (the motion-time curve showed "city wall"-like changes, and the anterior and posterior leaflets are moved in same direction during mid- and late diastole (see Fig. 3.23))?

- 2D echocardiography
  - Parasternal views:
    1. Is there annular calcification, and is this mild, moderate, or severe?
    2. Is there any thickening of the leaflets? Is this mild, moderate, or severe? Are both leaflets affected, and does this affect the tip or body of each leaflet?
    3. Is there any calcification of the leaflets? Is this focal or diffuse? Does the calcification affect either or both of the commissures?
    4. Is there fusion of one or both of the commissures?

Fig. 3.23 M-mode echocardiography shows a patient with rheumatic mitral stenosis. The mitral valves were thickened with "wall-like" change of the anterior and posterior leaflets moving in the same direction

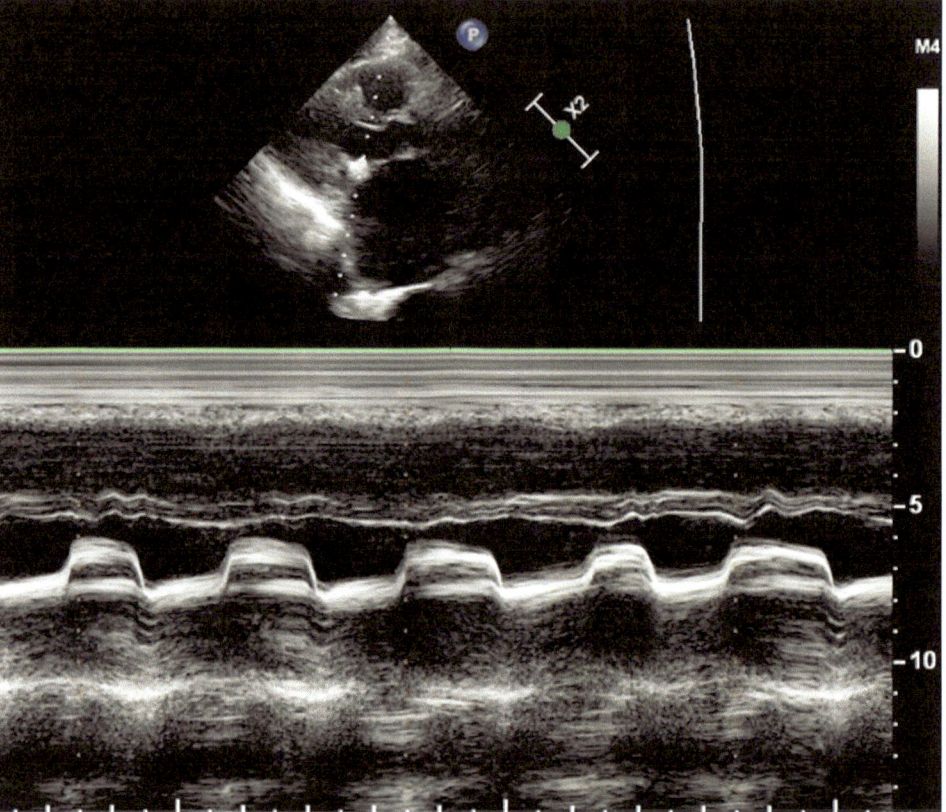

5. Is there any chordal thickening, shortening, or calcification? Does this affect the chordae to the anterior or posterior leaflet?

6. Is there any papillary muscles calcification or fibrosis?

7. Is mitral leaflet mobility reduced? Is it mild, moderate, or severe reduced? Is there any doming during diastole?

- If the image quality is good enough, the mitral orifice area should be measured in the parasternal short-axis view (mitral valve level). You should know stenosis mitral valve is funnel shaped, when open, so be careful to ensure that you are measuring the "funnel" at its narrowest point, i.e., the level of the leaflet tips.

- Apical views: The cardiac chamber size and function should be estimated from these views.

- Doppler echocardiography
  1. Use color Doppler to find any coexisting mitral regurgitation. Color jetting also helps to achieve proper alignment of the probes for CW and PW Doppler recording.
  2. Continuous Doppler: to measure the peak diastolic velocity of mitral valvular blood flow, and calculate the pressure gradient.
  3. From the trace of Doppler recording, measure the pressure half-time of the mitral valve inflow by measuring the downward slope of the E wave.

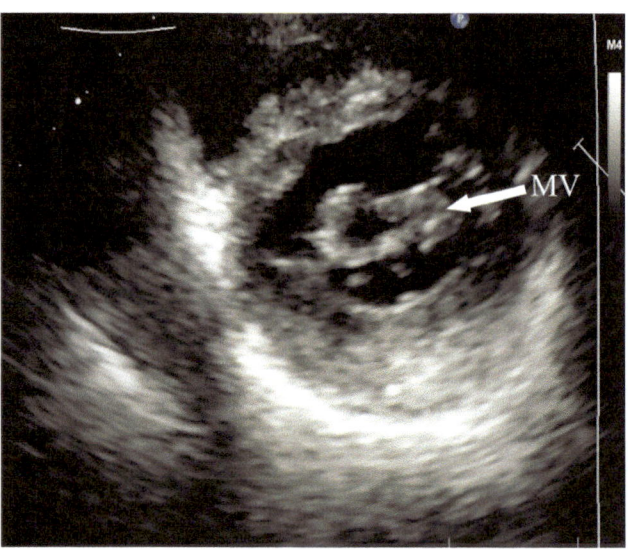

Fig. 3.24 2D echocardiography: Parasternal short-axis view shows that mitral valves (↑) were thickened with a "fish mouth" appearance during diastole

- 3D echocardiography

  It is helpful to observe the anatomical morphology, orifice and closing state of anterior and posterior mitral valve, subvalvular chordae tendineae and annulus more comprehensively and completely (Figs. 3.24, 3.25, 3.26, 3.27, and Table 3.2).

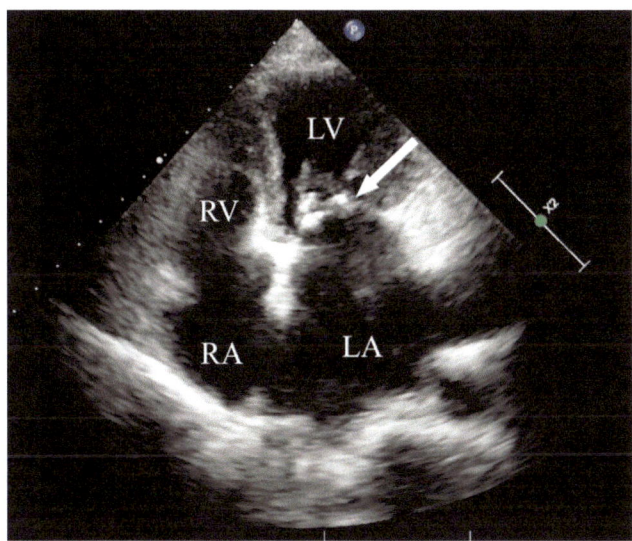

Fig. 3.25 2D echocardiography: Apical four-chamber view shows that both of anterior and posterior mitral leaflets (↑) were thickened with calcification

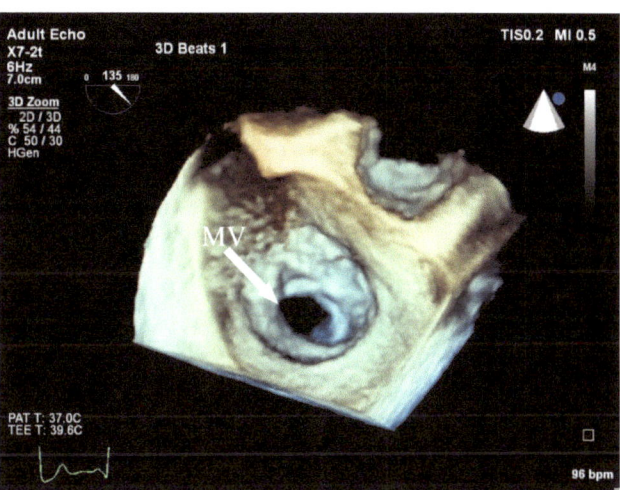

Fig. 3.27 3D echocardiography image from a patient with rheumatic mitral valve stenosis shows grossly thickened leaflets during diastole, giving a "fish mouth" (↑) appearance

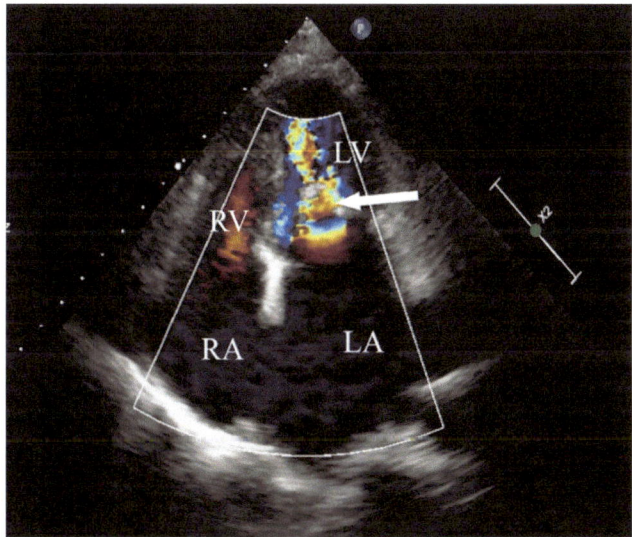

Fig. 3.26 Color Doppler echocardiography image shows the color flow (↑) of mitral valve blood with aliasing, which indicated the high velocity

Table 3.2 Indicators of mitral stenosis severity

	Mild	Moderate	Severe
Orifice area (cm²)	1.5–2.0	1.0–1.5	<1
Trans-mitral mean pressure gradient (mmHg)	<5	5–10	>10
Pulmonary artery systolic pressure (mmHg)	<30	30–50	>50

or aortic regurgitation can be relative indications. (3) Mitral stenosis with severe pulmonary hypertension, left ventricular too small, or patients with high risk of valve replacement surgery.

3.7.3 Echocardiography in Percutaneous Balloon Mitral Valvuloplasty

3.7.3.1 TEE for Guiding and Monitoring Percutaneous Balloon Mitral Valvuloplasty

On the basis of the four-chamber view of the middle esophagus (0–10°) and the short axis of the aortic valve (30–45°), the handle is rotated slightly to the right, and the double-chamber vein/double-atrial view of the middle esophagus (90–100°) can clearly show the overall appearance of the interatrial septum, and guide to select the appropriate inter-atrial puncture site.

The middle esophageal four-chamber view (0–10°), the mitral valve closure view (45–60°), two-chamber vein view (90°), aortic long-axis view (120–150°), and the short-axis view of the mitral valve of the gastric fundus are useful to

3.7.2 Pre-procedural TEE Screening for Mitral Stenosis: Mostly for Adult Acquired Rheumatic Mitral Stenosis

Indications: (1) moderate to severe mitral stenosis, no obvious deformation of the valve, good elasticity, no serious calcification, no obvious abnormality of the subvalvular structure, no thrombus in the left atrium, no moderate to severe mitral valvular regurgitation; (2) restenosis after surgery, atrial fibrillation, mitral calcification, and mild mitral

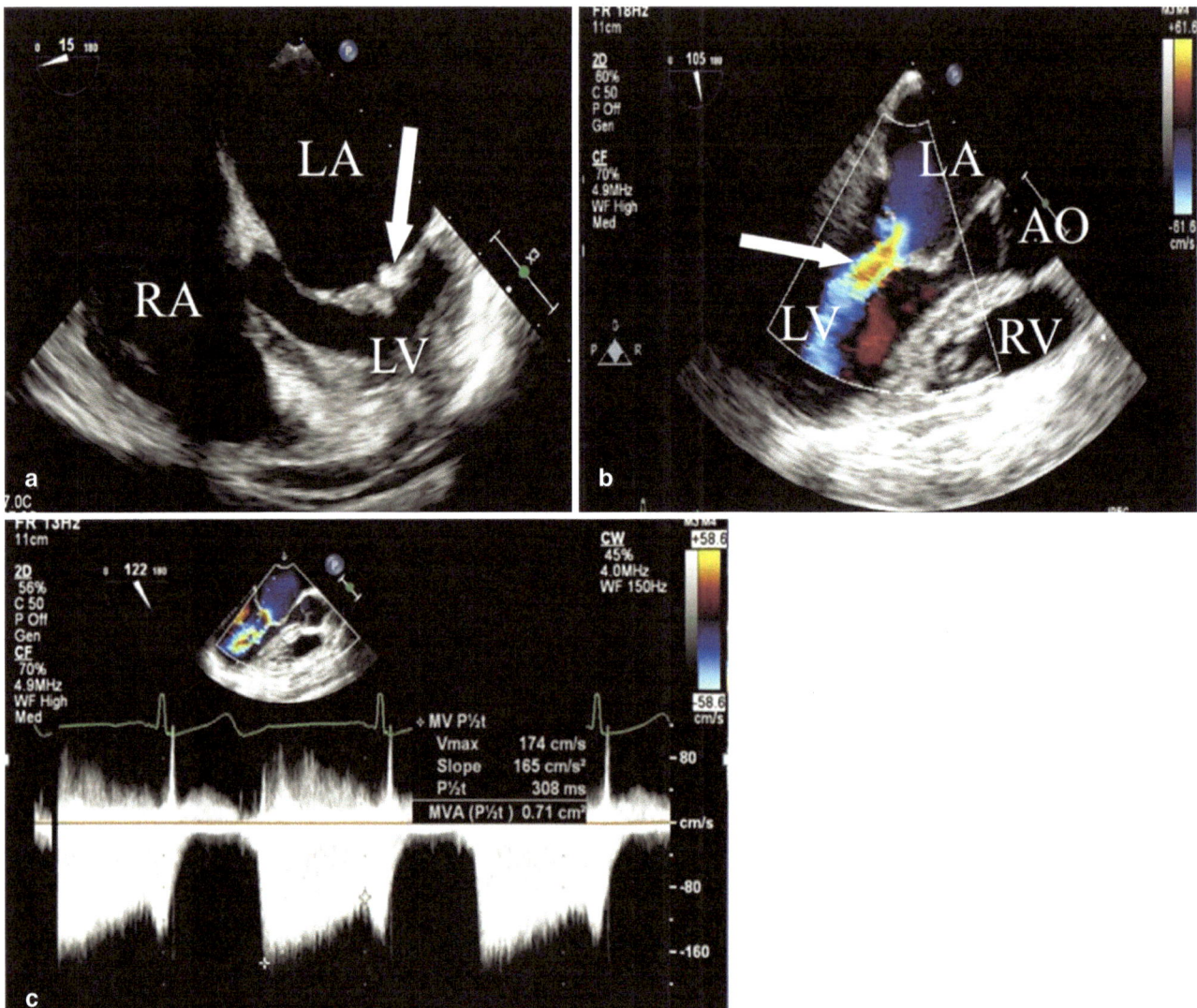

Fig. 3.28 (**a**) The four-chamber view of TEE image shows the thickened mitral valve (↑) with doming opening. (**b**) The four-chamber view with color Doppler of TEE image shows that the velocity of mitral inflow (↑) was high with aliasing. (**c**) Continues wave Doppler recording from same patient with mitral stenosis showed that the velocity of mitral inflow was high, the mitral valve orifice area was 0.7 cm² calculated by pressure half-time (PHT)

display the conditions of mitral valve and the chordae tendinous (see Figs. 3.28 and 3.29).

Percutaneous balloon mitral valvuloplasty (PBMV) is a technique in which a balloon is advanced to the heart via a femoral vein and a deliberate puncture is made in the interatrial septum to allow access to the left atrium. The balloon is then passed across the stenosis mitral valve and inflated to relieve the stenosis.

The technique works primarily through commissural splitting, and it is important to assess the mitral valve (and particularly the commissures) to select patients most likely to benefit from this procedure.

The procedural sequence should be monitored by TEE. The heart rate and blood pressure should be monitored during procedure. Following PBMV, assess the mitral valve carefully for any residual stenosis or for the regurgitation, and for any residual atrial septal defect.

The diastolic mitral orifice area, peak and mean transvalvular pressure should be measured to evaluate the improvement of mitral stenosis after valvuloplasty (Fig. 3.30). The pericardial effusion should be monitored during the procedure. If the mitral valve orifice area is >1.5 cm² and the degree of regurgitation is mild, the mitral valvuloplasty is successful.

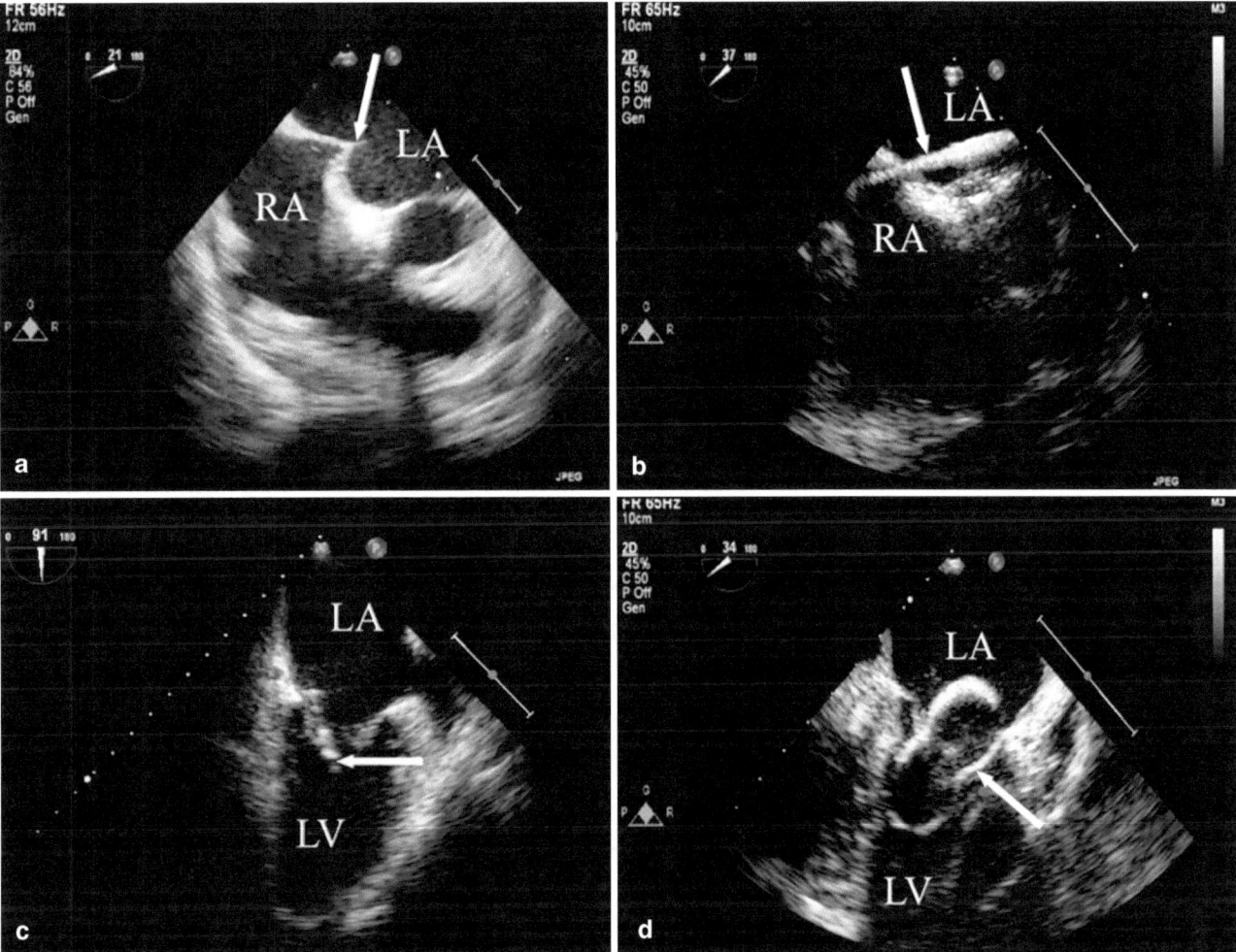

Fig. 3.29 Echocardiography-guided percutaneous mitral valvuloplasty. TEE images shows: (**a**) Catheter (↑) puncture atrial septum; (**b**) The balloon catheter (↑) was from the right atrium into the left atrium through the atrial septum; (**c**) The balloon catheter (↑) was through the mitral valve into the left ventricle; (**d**) The balloon catheter (↑) was passed through the stenosis mitral valve and the balloon was inflated to relieve the stenosis

3.7.3.2 TTE for Guiding and Monitoring Percutaneous Mitral Valvuloplasty

The parasternal short-axis view at the great artery level, the apical four-chamber view, and the subcostal double-atrium view are very useful for monitoring the sequence of mitral valvuloplasty. The indexes of observing before and after procedure and evaluating the effect of valvuloplasty are consistent with TEE guidance (see Fig. 3.31).

3.7.4 Echocardiographic Follow-Up After Mitral Stenosis Valvuloplasty

After mitral valvuloplasty, the patient should be followed up, and echocardiography examination should be performed at 24 h, 1 month, 3 months, 6 months, 1 year, and long term as needed

after valvuloplasty. The examination should focus on mitral valve orifice area, diastolic mitral forward flow velocity, mean transvalvular pressure gradient, mitral regurgitation, pulmonary systolic pressure, and the size and function of cardiac chamber.

3.8 Use of Echocardiography in Percutaneous Aortic Stenosis Valvuloplasty

3.8.1 Pre-procedural Echocardiographic Diagnosis of Congenital Aortic Stenosis

Aortic stenosis might be congenital or acquired. Congenital aortic stenosis is characterized by thickening, stiffness, and varying degrees of junctional fusion, resulting in narrowing

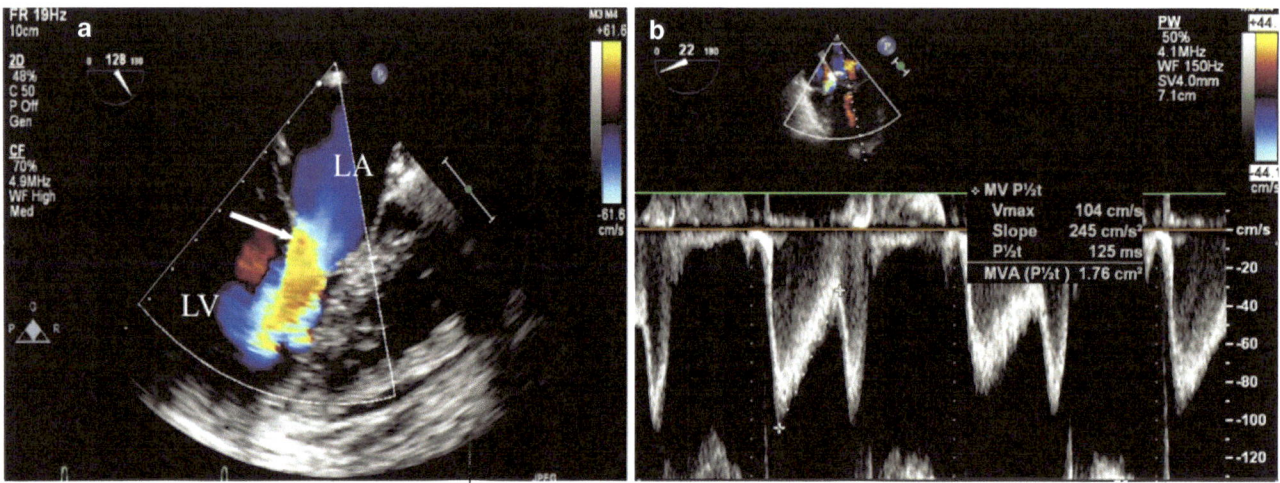

Fig. 3.30 (**a**) The TEE image with color Doppler recorded (↑) following valvuloplasty indicated that the mitral stenosis was improved. (**b**) Pulse Doppler tracing shows that the velocity of mitral diastolic blood flow was significantly decreased, and the area of mitral valve was about 1.8 cm² estimated by PHT after procedure

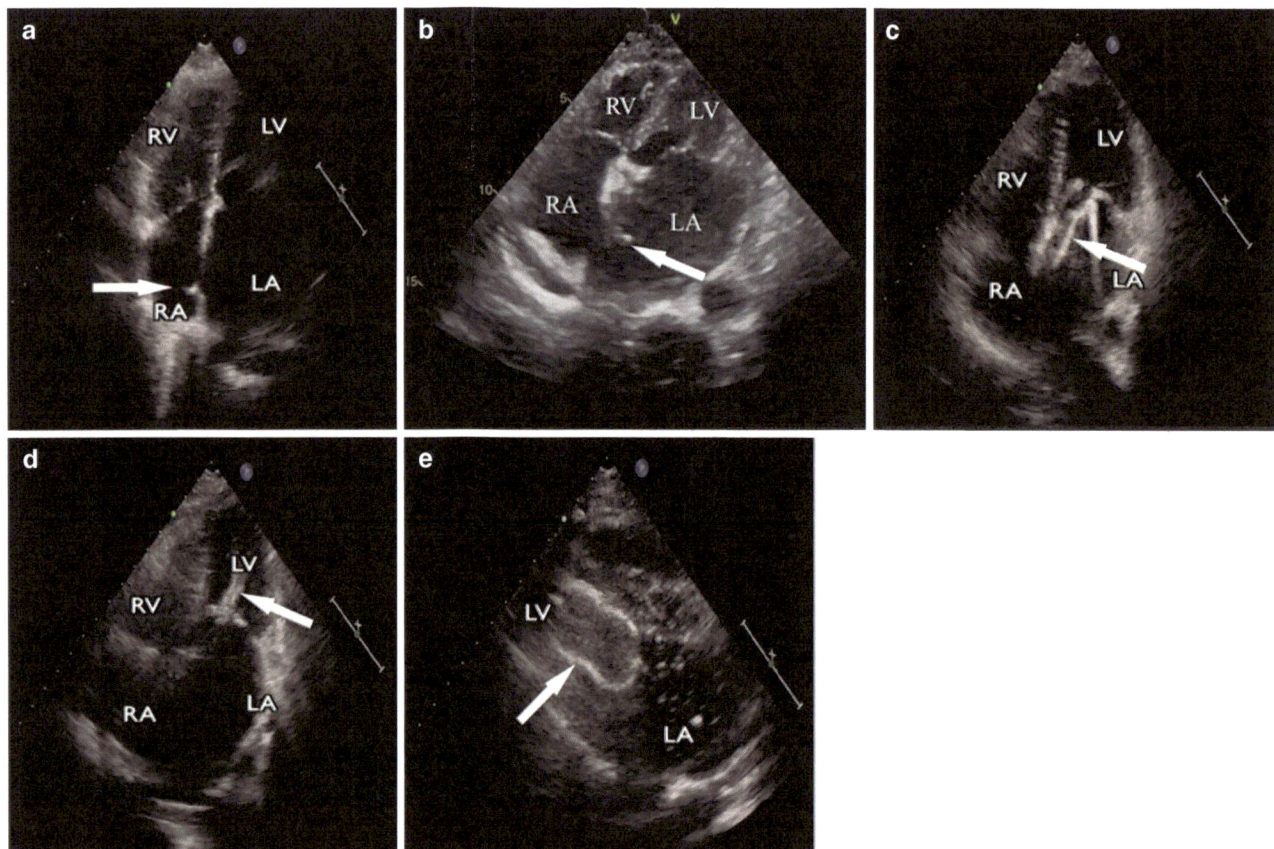

Fig. 3.31 Intraoperative TTE four-chamber images show: (**a**) the balloon catheter (↑) in the right atrium; (**b**) the catheter (↑) punctured the atrial septum; (**c**) the balloon catheter (↑) was in the left atrium; (**d**) the balloon catheter (↑) was passed through the stenosis mitral valve in the left ventricle; (**e**) after adjusting the position of the balloon catheter, the balloon (↑) was in the center of mitral valve orifice, and inflated

of the valve orifice. The number of aortic valves can be uni-, bi-, triple or quad leaflets, and congenital bicuspid aortic valve is the commonest congenital aortic valve abnormality. The prevalence of bicuspid aortic valve is 1–2% of the population, and it is thought to be responsible for around half of cases of severe aortic stenosis in adults.

- M-mode echocardiography: The echo density of aortic valve is enhanced and the valves are thickened (not obvious in children), and its motion curve of valvular opening is limited and the opening distance is reduced. The bicuspid aortic valve close line is eccentric.

- 2D echocardiography
  - **In the parasternal long- and short-axis (aortic valve level) views:**
    1. Assess the appearances and dimensions of the aortic valve (see Fig. 3.32). Fibrosis and calcification of a bicuspid aortic valve can distort the valve, lead to difficult recognition of its bicuspid nature on echocardiography.
    2. Look for evidence of cusp fusion (pseudo bicuspid valve)—the line where the cusps are fused is called a raphe. Describe which cusps are fused, valve thickness and calcification.

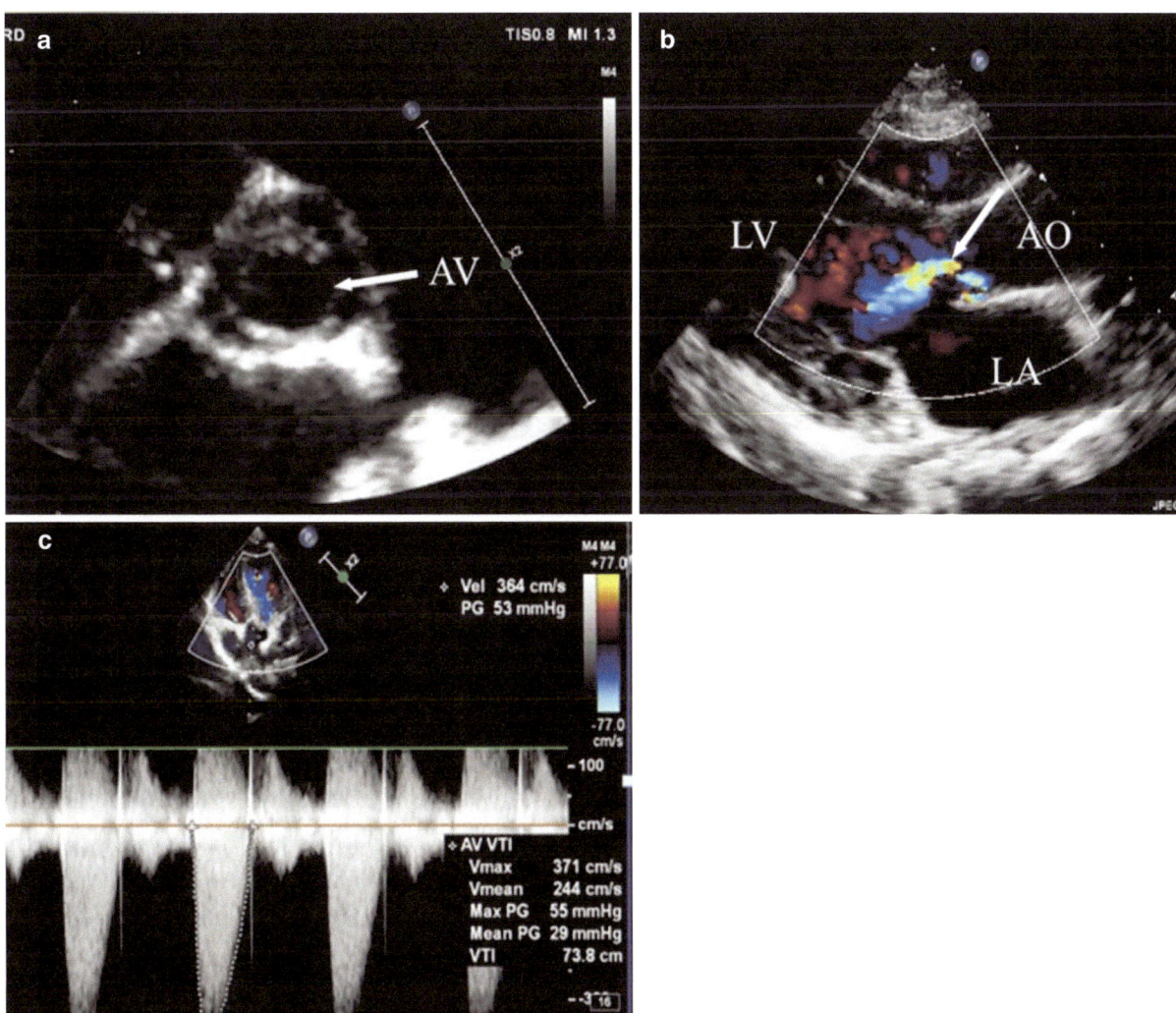

Fig. 3.32 TTE: (**a**) Parasternal short-axis view at the aortic valve level shows bicuspid aortic valve (↑) with anterior–posterior leaflets. The valves were mildly thickened. (**b**) Parasternal long-axis view with color Doppler shows that the velocity of blood flow through aortic valve was high. (**c**) Continuous Doppler tracing of aortic valve outflow shows that the peak velocity was 3.7 m/s, and peak pressure gradients was 55 mmHg

3. Assess aortic root dimensions, ascending aorta dilated after stenosis.
4. Assess left ventricular wall thickness and systole function.

- Doppler echocardiography
  1. The parasternal long-axis view and the apical five-chamber view with color Doppler can show the high velocity of blood flow through the stenotic aortic valve into the ascending aorta. Aortic valve regurgitation is seen in some patients.
  2. Use CW Doppler to assess flow through the aortic valve and assess the severity of any aortic stenosis or regurgitation.

3.8.2 Key Points on Echocardiographic Evaluation Before Balloon Dilatation for Aortic Stenosis

Indications: (1) Typical aortic stenosis without severe calcification; (2) Symptomatic congenital aortic valve stenosis; (3) The peak transvalvular gradient (>50 mmHg) is the intervention index; (4) Neonatal or infantile severe valvular stenosis, with congestive heart failure, can be used as a relief of symptoms, delayed surgery time; (5) Restenosis after surgical valvotomy.

3.8.3 Echocardiographic Guidance and Monitoring During Balloon Dilation for Aortic Stenosis

3.8.3.1 Procedure of Aortic Valvuloplasty Guided and Monitored Using TEE

The TEE probe was in mid esophagus at 30–45° showing short-axis view of aortic valve and at 120–150° showing long-axis view. Operator can observe the aortic valves clearly and assess the severity of stenosis or any regurgitation.

Before balloon dilatation, a temporary pacemaker electrode should be put into the right ventricular apex

guided by TEE. Percutaneous balloon aortic valvuloplasty is a technique in which a balloon is advanced to the heart via a femoral artery and access to the ascending aorta. The balloon is then passed through the stenotic aortic valve and inflated to relieve the stenosis. The technique works primarily through commissural splitting, and it is important to assess the aortic valve (and particularly the commissures) to select patients most likely to benefit from this procedure. The procedural sequence should be monitored by TEE. Before balloon inflation, operator should make sure that the temporary pacemaker is available. The heart rate, blood pressure, and pericardial effusion should be monitored during the procedure. It is generally believed that if the peak pressure gradient is reduced by more than 50% after inflation and the aortic regurgitation is mild, the procedure is successful.

3.8.3.2 Valvuloplasty Guided and Monitored by TTE

The aortic arch view from suprasternal fossa, parasternal short-axis view at great artery level, long-axis view, and the four-chamber view are very useful for monitoring the sequence of aortic valvuloplasty. The indexes of observing before and after procedure and evaluating the effect of valvuloplasty are consistent with TEE guidance (see Figs. 3.33 and 3.34).

3.8.4 Echocardiographic Assessment after Aortic Valvuloplasty

After aortic valvuloplasty, the patient should be followed up and echocardiography examination should be performed at 24 h, 1 month, 3 months, 6 months, 1 year, and long term as needed. The examination focuses on the velocity of aortic valve outflow, mean transvalvular pressure gradient, aortic valve and peri-valve regurgitation, the left ventricular size, function and wall thickness.

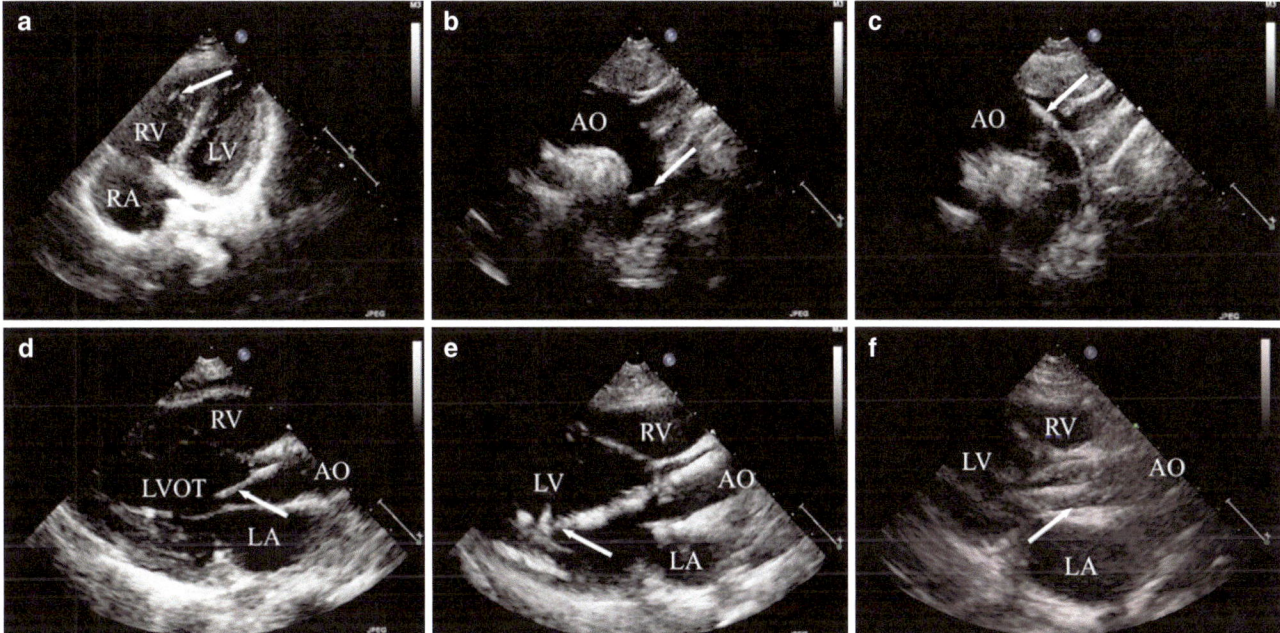

Fig. 3.33 TTE images: (**a**) apical four-chamber view shows the tip of pace maker electrode (↑) in the right ventricle apex. (**b**) The aortic arch view from suprasternal fossa window shows the balloon catheter (↑) in the descending aorta. (**c**) The aortic arch view shows the balloon catheter (↑) in the ascending aorta. (**d**) The parasternal long-axis view shows that the balloon catheter (↑) crosses the aortic valve into left ventricular outflow tract. (**e**) The same view shows that the balloon catheter (↑) enters the left ventricle; (**f**) The balloon (↑) is passing through the aortic valve orifice

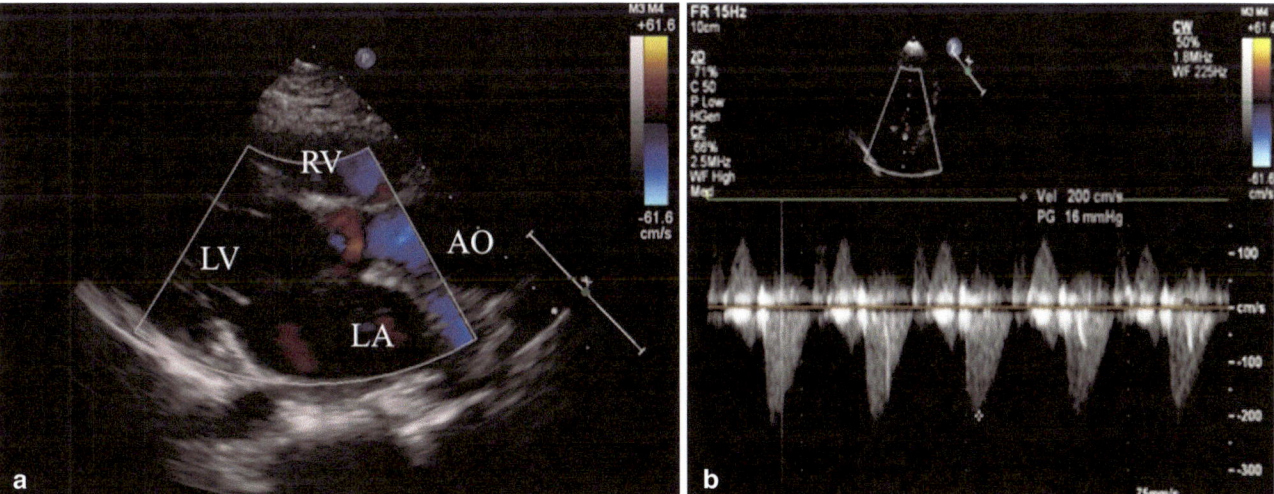

Fig. 3.34 The improvement of aortic stenosis and regurgitation was evaluated after each balloon expansion. (**a**) Color Doppler shows that the color flow of aortic valve was improved and a small amount of sys-tolic regurgitation; (**b**) Continuous Doppler shows that systolic blood flow velocity was significantly reduced, peak pressure gradient was about 23 mmHg

Atrial septal defect (ASD) occurs in an estimated 0.67% of live births and 6–10% of individuals with congenital heart disease. The sex ratio is 1:2–1:3, and it is more common among females. This chapter describes percutaneous interventional closure of ostium secundum ASD, which accounts for 80% of ASD, with ostium primum and sinus venosus ASD accounting for 10%, respectively. This chapter introduces how to perform PAN procedure for ASD and PFO.

Closure via femoral vein approach using an occluder delivered through a delivery sheath is successful in about 80% of ostium secundum ASDs. Since King et al. first introduced percutaneous ASD closure in 1976, development and improvement of devices and techniques along with wide use, the incidence of complications has decreased to a very low level with favorable long-term outcomes.

4.1 Anatomical Features

There is great variation in position and diameter of ostium secundum ASD, from 2 to 3 mm to complete defect in atrial septum or a sieve mesh appearance. In general, ostium secundum ASD is divided into the following four types according to defect position:

1. Central or oval foramen type is the most common (75% of cases), located at the center of atrial septum with normal structure surrounding. Coronary sinus lay below and anterior to the defect. Most can be treated by percutaneous closure.
2. Inferior vena cava type is also common (15% of cases), generally large and located posteriorly, and usually not amenable to percutaneous closure because it connects

with the inferior vena cava entrance without or with a thin film atrial septal edge.
3. Superior vena cava or sinus venosus type (4% of cases) is located posterosuperiorly at the connection between superior vena cava and right atrium and always accompanied by anomalous right superior pulmonary venous connection. In general, patch repair is performed with extracorporeal circulation.
4. Mixed type has the latter two or more deformities, accounts for 6% of cases, spans most of the atrial septum, and is treated usually by patch repair with extracorporeal circulation.

4.2 Pathophysiology

Because the left ventricle is less compliant than the right ventricle, left atrial pressure is 3–5 mmHg higher than right atrial pressure. Therefore, ASD manifests with left-to-right shunt with volume depending on ASD size and left and right ventricular compliance. In small ASD, which sometimes can be found in routine echocardiographic examination, the shunt volume is small without obvious symptoms and signs. If the ASD is large, the pulmonary circulation flow will be up to 1.5 times the systemic circulation flow. With more blood getting through the right heart system, the right atrium and ventricle, and the pulmonary trunk enlarges, while the left atrium and ventricle shrink, and the aortic diameter decreases. A large left-to-right shunt causes pulmonary arteriolar spasm. With increasing age, intimal hyperplasia and media thickening gradually cause vessel stenosis, and increased resistance leads to pulmonary artery hypertension, which in turn reduces volume from left to right shunt and causes right atrium and ventricle hypertrophy. After the right heart system pressure increases to some extent, some bloodstream may deviate to the left atrium generating Eisenmenger's syndrome. Cyanosis is a manifestation of late phases of the disease.

Electronic Supplementary Material The online version of this chapter (https://doi.org/10.1007/978-981-15-2055-6_4) contains supplementary material, which is available to authorized users.

4.3   Indications and Contraindications for ASD Closure

1. Indications
   - Age ≥1 year old.
   - Central type defect, diameter ≥5 mm with right heart volume overload.
   - ≥5 mm distance from defect edge to coronary sinus, and superior and inferior vena cava, and ≥7 mm distance from defect edge to atrioventricular valve [1].
   - Atrial septum diameter is larger than the selected occluder diameter at the left atrium.
   - Defects with well-defined margins except aortic side.
2. Contraindications
   - Ostium primum or sinus venosus ASD.
   - Endocarditis and hemorrhagic diseases.
   - Thrombus presence at occluder location or at catheter insertion site.
   - Severe pulmonary artery hypertension with right-to-left shunt.
   - Severe myocarditis or valvular diseases unrelated to ASD.
   - Infectious diseases within 1 month or uncontrolled infection.
   - Other heart deformity requiring surgical treatment.

4.4   Patent Foramen Ovale

Patent foramen ovale (PFO) is a physiological channel of cardiac atrial septum in embryonic period. Most primary septum and secondary septum will fuse together to form intact atrial septum. The PFO is formed in the absence of fusion. PFO has long been considered to have no obvious clinical significance. However, with the development of imaging technology, echocardiography clearly shows the long thrombus of PFO, which makes the relationship between PFO and stroke and systemic embolism widely concerned. Most PFO do not require treatment. However, the blood clot may enter the left heart from the right heart, thereby entering the systemic circulation, resulting in arterial embolization. This phenomenon of thrombosis or chemical embolism through special channels is called paradoxical embolism. A stroke or transient ischemic attack occurs if cerebral artery embolized. The patients with PFO combined with paradoxical embolism are recommended to be treated with occlusion and interventional method, postoperative treatment, and complications are same as ASD.

The primary atrial septum is fibrous tissue, which is thin and wiggling. The secondary septum is thicker muscular tissue. The degree of overlap between primary and secondary septum is the length of PFO, and the distance of non-fusion is the width and size of PFO. The length range of PFO is 3 ~ 18 mm, average 8 mm, width range 1 ~ 19 mm, average 4.9 mm, and its size increases with age.

In normal people, left atrial pressure is 3 ~ 5 mmHg higher than that of right atrium. PFO is closed and cause no blood shunting. When chronic or transient pressure in the right atrium is increased beyond the left atrium, the weak primary septum in the left side is pushed away, showing right to left shunt [2].

Indications

1. Age > 16 years old (age can be appropriately relaxed if there is clear evidence of paradoxical embolism).
2. PFO with unexplained stroke or transient ischemic attack (TIA).
3. PFO associated with cerebral infarction/TIA, patients with definite deep venous thrombosis or pulmonary embolism is not suitable for anticoagulant therapy.
4. PFO associated with cerebral infarction/TIA, which is still recurrent with antiplatelet or anticoagulant therapy.
5. Stroke or peripheral embolism due to unknown cause combined with PFO and right heart or implants surface have thrombosis.

Contraindications

1. Cerebral embolism with a clear cause.
2. Contraindications for antiplatelet or anticoagulation therapy, such as severe bleeding within 3 months, obvious retinopathy, other history of intracranial hemorrhage, and obvious intracranial diseases.
3. Thrombosis of the inferior vena cava or pelvic vein results in complete obstruction, systemic or local infection, sepsis, and intracardiac thrombosis.
4. Combined pulmonary hypertension or PFO is a special channel.
5. Massive cerebral infarction within 4 weeks.

4.5   Pre-procedural Preparation

1. Routine laboratory examinations include routine hematology testing and blood type, biochemical testing, coagulation function, viral hepatitis and other infectious diseases, electrocardiography, chest radiography, and echocardiography.
2. Pre-procedural blood preparation, skin preparation, fasting of solids and liquids, and peripheral superficial vein access.
3. Procedural plan and possible risks and complications are communicated to patients and their families with verification of their understanding and approval. The procedure can be performed only after families sign an informed consent form.

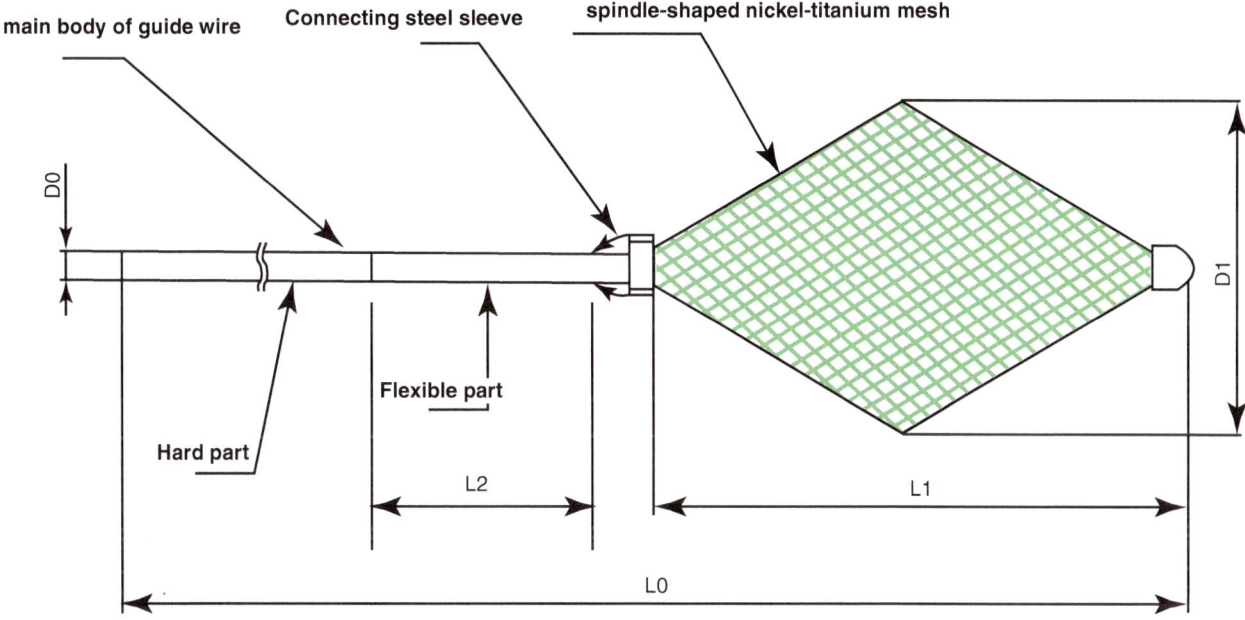

Fig. 4.1 Schematic diagram of the Novel echocardiographic guide wire (Panna™ wire)

4. Device preparation
   - Occluder: Currently available and commonly used occluders have a two-sided discoid structure. There are several brands and types of domestic occluders approved by the China Food and Drug Administration. For instance, with the occluder from Shanghai Shape Memory Alloy Co., Ltd., type and size are determined according to waist diameter which ranges from 6 to 40 mm at 2 mm intervals.
   - Arterial sheath: If child's weight is ≤12 kg, a 6F arterial sheath for upper limb is prepared; if >12 kg, a 7F arterial sheath for lower extremity is prepared.
   - 6F multipurpose catheter (Cordis, 100 cm, 0.038 in. [0.965 mm])
   - Super-stiff guide wire (Cook's Lunderquist, 260 cm, 0.038 in. [0.965 mm])
   - Delivery sheath: 8F, 9F, 10F, 12F, and 14F delivery sheaths are recommended for 6–12 mm, 14–16 mm, 18–24 mm, 26–30 mm, and 32–40 mm occluders, respectively.
   - The novel echocardiography-guided wire: The novel guide wire, which is specialized for echocardiography guidance, is made of a high-strength nickel-titanium material, with a spindle-shaped nickel-titanium alloy mesh at the tip. The guide wire consists of two portions: stiff and flexible portion, which is welded together with the spindle mesh by steel sleeve. Nitinol material is used for the main body of guide wire and spindle-shaped nickel-titanium mesh, and 316LV stainless steel is used for steel sleeve

(Fig. 4.1). The spindle-shaped tip section is easily detected under echocardiography during the procedure due to large cross section and spindle-shaped. Therefore, it is recommended to use an echocardiography-guided wire instead of the super-stiff guide wire for beginners.

4.6 Procedure

4.6.1 TTE-Guided Interventional Closure of ASD via Femoral Vein Approach (Fig. 4.2)

The procedure can be performed in a general cardiac operating room, cardiac catheterization room or outpatient operating room. Adults and older children who can cooperate should receive local anesthesia and sedatives; infants and young children must undergo general anesthesia with spontaneous breathing. The distance between the third intercostal space at right midclavicular line and the puncture site in right femoral vein (or the left if right femoral vein puncture fails) is measured and marked on the catheter and guide wire as working length. A sterile drape is placed between umbilical level and patient's knees. After femoral vein puncture, an arterial sheath is inserted, and heparin 80 U/kg is administered.

The 6F multipurpose catheter and super-stiff guide wire are delivered through the arterial sheath. The head of the super-stiff guide wire should be extend 2–4 cm outside the

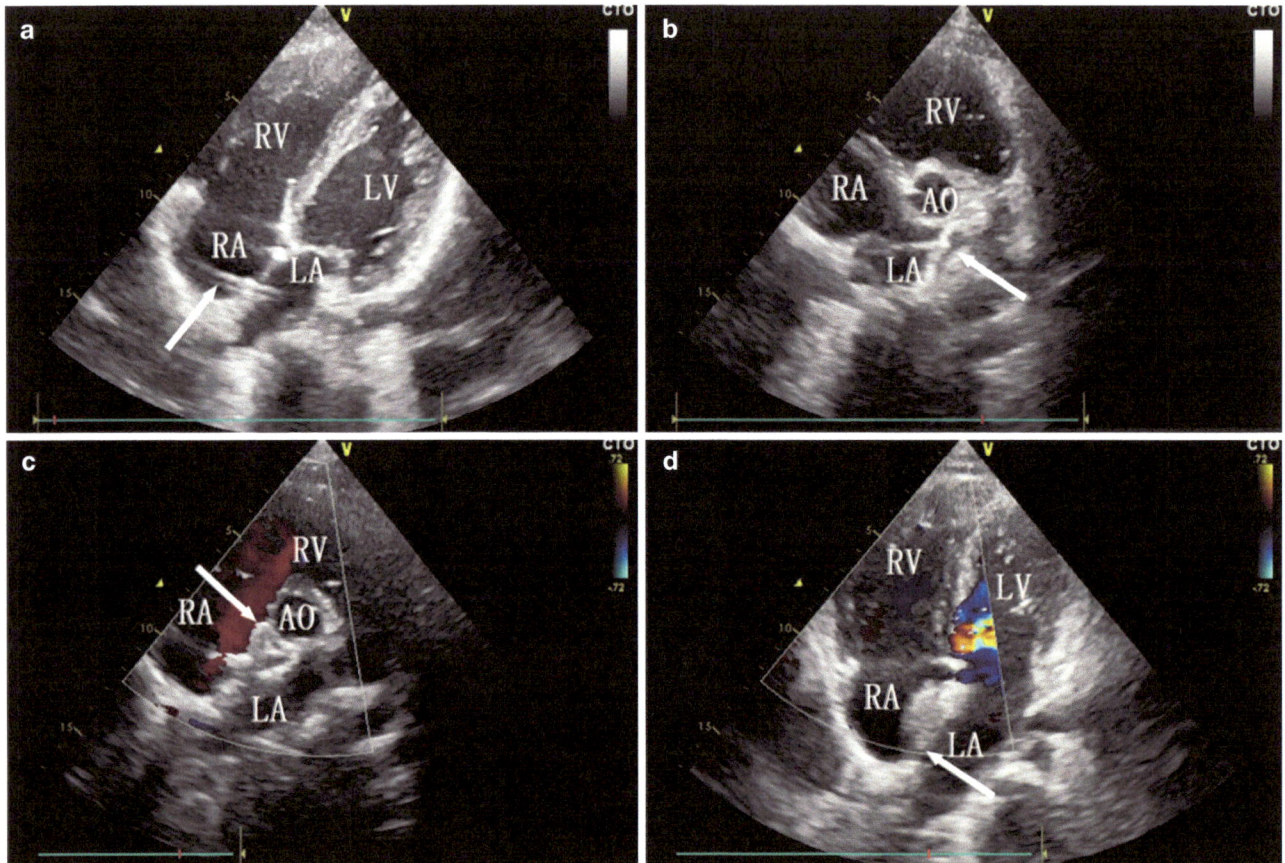

Fig. 4.2 TTE-guided interventional closure of ASD by femoral vein approach. (**a**) Apical four-chamber view shows the delivery sheath (↑) crosses ASD. (**b**) Parasternal short-axis view shows the occluder (↑) is released in left atrium. (**c**) Parasternal short-axis view shows the occluder (↑) is released in both sides of atrial septum. (**d**) Apical four-chamber view shows the occluder (↑) is completely released in good position. *LA* Left atrium, *RA* Right atrium, *LV* Left ventricle, *RV* Right ventricle, *AO* Aorta

catheter, and push the catheter and the guide wire as one unit. If there is obvious resistance, the catheter and guide wire should be withdrawn back into the arterial sheath. And fix the catheter, re-push the guide wire and try again, and avoid pushing the catheter violently. The acoustic shadow of the catheter and guide wire can be detected in the inferior vena cava in the subcostal long-axis view while pushing the catheter. After inserting the catheter and guide wire in the vein to working length, withdraw the guide wire and rotate the catheter clockwise gently. The catheter can be positioned using apical four-chamber view. The operator should adjust the catheter orientation under TTE guidance and insert it through the ASD to the left atrium; be careful to avoid deep insertion and damaging the left atrium wall. A small amount of normal saline can be injected through the catheter to confirm it position. The guide wire is inserted through the catheter to a depth that does not exceed 5–7 cm than the working length. After the guide wire and catheter are inserted to the marked depth, withdraw the catheter and marked the depth on the catheter, and left the guide wire in position, and then remove the arterial sheath, insert a delivery sheath into the left atrium through guide wire. The insertion depth should be consistent with the catheter insertion depth described above. When the guide wire and the core of the delivery sheath are removed, the outer sheath should be inserted and kept the proximal end of the delivery sheath in the left atrium. The occluder size should be selected by adding 4–6 mm to the maximum diameter of the ASD measured by the TTE. The length of the atrial septum is measured to determine if the occluder can be fully opened. For large ASD or thin defect edges, the occluder diameter can be increased by 8–10 mm. Under TTE monitoring, the catheter of the ASD closed system should be filled with normal saline to avoid sucking in air due to negative pressure during the procedure.

After successful placement of the occluder, the position of the occluder, the effects on surrounding structures such as the mitral valve, pulmonary veins and coronary sinus and residual shunt should be observed in the aortic short-axis, apical four-chamber and subcostal views. The occluder is released after confirmation of the non-interference with the surrounding structures, the delivery system is removed, the puncture site is sutured and bandage; pressure bandage is used to stop bleeding, and the patient is directly transferred to the general ward after waking up [3, 4].

4.6.2 TEE-Guided Interventional ASD Closure via Femoral Vein Approach (Fig. 4.3)

The procedure is performed in a general cardiac operating room or cardiac catheterization laboratory. The patient underwent general anesthesia, endotracheal intubation, and a transesophageal echocardiographic probe is placed into esophagus. The distance between the third intercostal space at right midclavicular line and the puncture site in right femoral vein is measured and marked on the catheter and guide wire during procedure. A sterile drape is placed between umbilical level and patient's knees. The size of the occluder was chosen by adding 4–6 mm to the ASD maximum diameter measured by TEE, and the total length of atrial septum is measured to determine if the occluder can be completely opened. Occluder diameter may be increased by 8–10 mm for large ASD or thin defect edge. The occluder is soaked in heparin saline and then is placed in a loading sheath. After systemic heparinization (80 U/kg), puncture the right femoral vein and place the arterial sheath. The 6F multipurpose catheter and super-stiff guide wire are delivered through the arterial sheath. After reaching the working length, the TEE can detect the catheter, which advances through the inferior vena cava into the right atrium in the bilateral atrial view, and send the catheter and guide wire through the ASD under echocardiography guidance. Withdrawn the inner core of delivery sheath and the arterial sheath. Then, an occluder is delivered carefully through the delivery sheath (Fig. 4.3). The limited exposure range of esophageal echocardiographic field in some patients, TTE parasternal short-axis view at aortic valve level is preferred and more convenient. The TEE double-atrium view is better than TTE to assess deployment process and occluder position more clearly. After successful placement of the occluder, the position of the occlude, the effects on surrounding structures such as the mitral valve, pulmonary veins and coronary sinus and residual shunt should be observed in the aortic short-axis, apical four-chamber and subcostal views. If the position of the occluder and the mitral valve, the pulmonary veins and the coronary sinus function are well, the occluder is released.

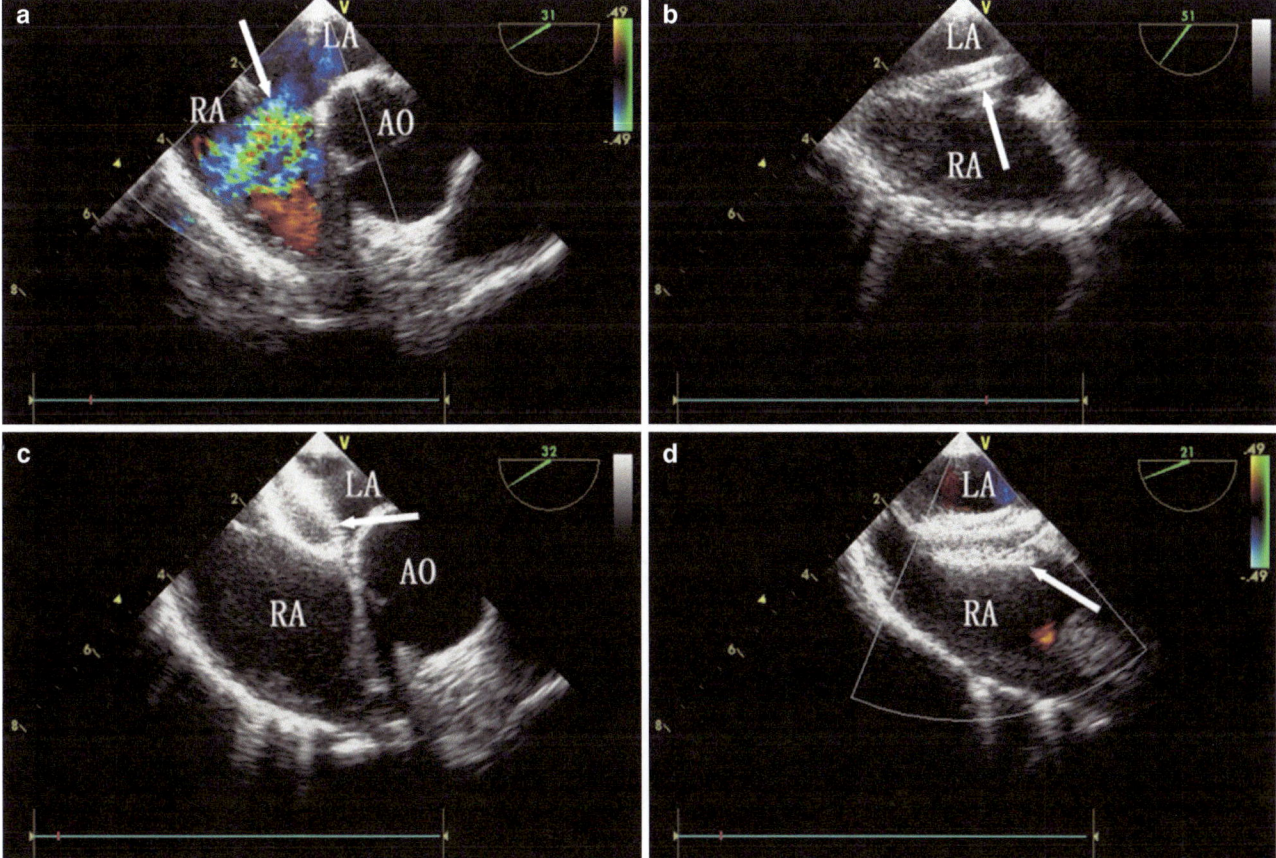

Fig. 4.3 TEE-guided interventional closure of ASD by femoral vein approach. (**a**) Short-axis view with color Doppler shows the shunt of ASD (↑) and tricuspid regurgitation. (**b**) Short-axis view shows the delivery sheath (↑) crossing ASD. (**c**) TEE short-axis view shows the disk of occluder (↑) is released in left atrial side. (**d**) The TEE double-atrium view shows the occluder (↑) is completely released and in good position. *LA* Left atrium, *RA* Right atrium, *AO* Aorta

The delivery system is removed, the puncture site is sutured and bandage; pressure bandage is used to stop bleeding. Patients should be extubated in operating room or intensive care unit, and transferred to a general ward after stabilization [5].

4.7   Post-procedural Management

Post procedure, the sandbag is pressed at puncture site for 4 h and the patient should remain in supine position for 12 h. Antibiotics are given intravenously once half an hour pre-procedure and 6h post-procedure, low-molecular weight heparin is administered subcutaneously 24 h post-procedure. For adults with occluder diameter ≥30 mm, clopidogrel 75 mg/day can be administered; for patients with atrial fibrillation, warfarin should be administered indefinitely.

4.8   Complications and Treatment

4.8.1   Complications of Cardiac Procedures Without Extracorporeal Circulation

These include anesthesia-related complication and infective endocarditis.

4.8.2   Occluder Displacement and Migration

Intraprocedural displacement is mainly related to cable rotation, loose occluder screw, and other factors. Occluder displacement, with an incidence of about 0.24–1.44%, is mainly related to thin, soft and short edge of ASD or false choose of smaller occluder. The occluder can migrate into either atrium (usually to right atrium) and subsequently enter the right or left ventricle, and even the pulmonary or systemic circulation. When occluder displacement occurs, patients may experience palpitations, chest pain, arrhythmia, and other symptoms. Echocardiographic evaluation before and during procedure is therefore most important. If the TTE window is unclear or the defect is large, TEE should be used to further assess defect edge status. Especially for patients with thin inferior vena cava edge, occluder should be pushed repeatedly and its shape and location confirmed using the parasternal short-axis view at aortic valve level, and apical four-chamber and subcostal views before occluder release. Intraoperative operation should be standardized, and appropriate occluder should be selected, especially the patients with thin and short edge of the inferior vena cava. Before releasing the occluder, it is necessary to repeatedly push and pull the occluder under the short axis of the aorta and the apex views guidance. The shape and position of the occluder should be confirmed by subcostal views. If the occluder is detached during the operation, you can try to catch the occluder with a snare and pull it out through a larger sheath. For most patients, conventional surgery should be performed immediately.

4.8.3   Residual Shunt

At early stages, dotted shunts may appear within occluder but without separated blood flow. Residual shunt severity is defined according to the diameter of left-to-right shunt as: if <1 mm is trivial; if 1–2 mm is mild; if 2–4 mm is moderate; and if >4 mm is severe. The incidence of immediate residual shunt is 6–40%, in contrast to 4–12% 72 h post procedure, and only 0.1–5% after 3 months. Residual shunt mainly occurs in slender, oval defects when occluder opens but its edge does not closely fit the defect; or if the defect has multiple holes or sieve pores, residual shunt may occur after closing the larger but not the smaller defects. In general, a residual shunt through the occluder will not be treated because endothelialization will close it; however, there should be no hemolysis. If a >5 mm shunt is found beyond the occluder coverage area, deploying another occluder to ensure complete closure should be considered; If the defect is less than 5 mm, it can be temporarily not treated.

4.8.4   Arrhythmia

During the operation, due to the stimulation of the heart by procedure, various arrhythmias often occur, including supraventricular tachycardia, sinus bradycardia and ventricular premature beats. Generally, no special treatment is needed, and the heart rhythm will be restored after stopping the stimulation. After occluder placement, atrioventricular node and surrounding tissues might be fricative and cause temporary edema of these tissue and lead to atrioventricular node dysfunction or failure, and hemodynamic change may have negative effect on the electrophysiological properties of cardiac tissues. Patients may develop sinus bradycardia, atrioventricular block, atrial or ventricular premature beats with an incidence of 2–4%. Although post-procedural arrhythmia is usually transient, it may last for several hours or even longer in some patients. Therefore, within 3 months after ASD closure, care should be taken to avoid strenuous activity and reduce the stimulation of the surrounding tissue by the occluder. In case of conduction block, temporary or permanent pacemaker treatment may be placed if necessary, and in some patients, arrhythmia will disappear after removal of the occluder.

4.8.5 Headache or Migraine

The incidence rate is about 7%, the performance of pain varies from person to person, some with nausea, vomiting, tinnitus, hearing loss or limb numbness; mostly occurs when the occluder has chosen that its surface cannot form intact endothelialization, or Insufficient antiplatelet therapy or aspirin resistance, resulting in microthrombus formation and shedding, obstructing cerebral blood vessels. Therefore, antiplatelet therapy after ASD interventional therapy for at least half a year, for patients with occlusion device diameter greater than 30 mm, or symptomatic, should decide whether to add clopidogrel to strengthen antiplatelet therapy or switch to warfarin anticoagulation according to the condition.

4.8.6 Occluder Erosion

This is a severe complications of ASD closure, the incidence rate is about 0.1–0.5%, such as aortic-right atrial fistula, patients may have heart continuous murmur; if the occluder erodes outwards the heart, the patient may have pericardial effusion. The reason maybe that the defect edge is short and the occluder is too large, and the aorta and atrial wall were fricated by the inserted occluder, so the indication should be strictly controlled. Once the above complications occur, the occluder should usually be surgically removed and treated accordingly.

4.8.7 Hemorrhage or Thromboembolism

Hemorrhage includes gastrointestinal tract and cerebral bleeding. Thrombus, which always forms on the occluder left atrial surface may lead to systemic thromboembolism, including peripheral and retinal arterial thromboembolism. In China, reported incidence of thromboembolism is low, and it can be further reduced by systematically and rationally using heparin and antiplatelet drugs during and after procedure according to patient risk profile. For large diameter ASD, echocardiographic follow-up at 6 months after closure allows to timely detect possible thrombus on the occluder surface. Anticoagulation therapy should be continued and increased in dosing, if thrombus is found. If thrombus is large, surgery should be considered to minimize embolization risk. Thrombosis occurs mostly on the left atrial surface of the occluder, which can cause systemic thromboembolism, such as peripheral arterial embolization, retinal arterial embolization, etc. Heparin and antiplatelet agents should be used reasonably during perioperative period, and individualized treatment should be performed according to the patient's situation.

Anticoagulant drugs should be discontinued and symptomatic treatment should be carried out in case of hemorrhagic manifestations.

4.8.8 Hemolysis

Hemolysis is a rare complication and most commonly secondary to damage to red blood cells flowing through the occluder. If urine becomes dark brown or progressive anemia develops, aspirin and other antiplatelet drugs should be discontinued to promote thrombus formation on the occluder surface. Large doses of glucocorticoids should be performed to stabilize cell membranes and reduce cell fragmentation.

4.9 Cases

Case 1 TTE-guided interventional closure via femoral vein approach of typical ASD (Video 4.1).

Presentation: A 34-year-old man weighing 68 kg and with 99% SPO_2 in all limbs was admitted to hospital for a murmur that had been found during physical examination 1 week ago. The patient had frequent colds and fatigue when he was a child, but no cyanosis. ECG showed sinus rhythm and chest X-ray showed congenital heart disease with increased pulmonary circulation. Echocardiography with clear window showed an ASD (13 × 9 mm², central), all edges >7 mm. Left ventricular end diastolic diameter was 45 mm and ejection fraction was 63%.

Analysis: The patient was 34 years old and could be cooperated during operation. Preoperative transthoracic echocardiography showed the patient has good echocardiographic windows. Decision was made to treat ASD by TTE-guided interventional closure via femoral vein approach using conscious sedation.

Procedure: Procedure was performed in a general cardiac operating room using conscious sedation. The distance between the third intercostal space at right midclavicular line and the puncture site in right femoral vein was measured and marked on the catheter and guide wire as the working length. A sterile drape was placed between umbilical level and patient's knees. After systemic heparinization (80 U/kg), right femoral vein puncture was carried out. A sheath was inserted, and a 6F multipurpose catheter and super-stiff guide wire were advanced through an arterial sheath via the inferior vena cava into the right atrium through ASD in the middle of atrial septum under the guidance of echocardiography. The catheter and sheath then were withdrawn, and a 12F delivery sheath was advanced to left atrium along super-stiff guide wire. After guide wire and delivery sheath core withdrawal, a 22 mm ASD occluder was advanced under TTE monitoring for closure. After successfully implantation, parasternal short-axis view at aortic valve level, and apical four-chamber and sub-xiphoid views by TTE confirmed that occluder did not affect mitral valve, pulmonary vein, coronary sinus, or adjacent cardiac structure. Compression bandages were applied after pulling out the delivery sheath and stitching the puncture site. Patient was transferred to a general ward.

Case 2 TTE-guided interventional closure via femoral vein approach of large type ASD with aortic edge insufficiency (Video 4.2).

Presentation: A 3.5-year-old boy weighing 15 kg and containing 99% SPO_2 in all limbs was admitted to hospital for the murmurs found during the physical examination 2 years ago. ECG showed sinus rhythm, enlarged right atrium and ventricle, and incomplete right bundle branch block. In chest X-ray, right atrium and ventricle and pulmonary artery were enlarged with increased pulmonary flow, suggesting an ASD. Echocardiography image showed an ASD (13 mm, central) without an aortic side edge, and other edges >7 mm. Left ventricular end diastolic diameter was 30 mm and ejection fraction was 63%.

Analysis: The ASD with 13 mm defect met indications for percutaneous interventional closure. Aortic side had no edge and others were greater than 7 mm. A adjustable curved sheath was prepared because the defect was large and without an aortic side edge.

Procedure: Procedure was performed in a general cardiac operating room under general anesthesia. The distance between the third intercostal at right midclavicular line and the puncture site in right femoral vein was measured and marked on the catheter and guide wire as the working length. The femoral vein was punctured, heparin was given, and a 6 French multipurpose catheter with a super-stiff wire was advanced to cross the defect. After crossing the defect and obtaining a safe and stable position of the catheter on the left side of the heart, multipurpose catheter was withdrawn. The size of the occluder was chosen by adding 4–6 mm to the ASD maximum diameter measured by transthoracic echocardiography. Once the device had been chosen, the delivery sheath was advanced over the super-stiff wire into the left atrium. The wire and the core were removed very slowly from the delivery sheath, positioned in a lower position, allowing free flow of blood coming out from the sheath, in order to reduce the risk of air embolism. When placing occluder by routine method, the occluder fell into right atrium several times, and pulmonary vein release technique was used. The device was advanced into the delivery sheath to deploy the left disc partially in the left supra pulmonary vein, then the sheath was pulled back in the right atrium allowing the right disc of the device to be deployed in the right atrium, and the left disc would be deployed simultaneously in left atrium. The correct device position was assessed by echocardiography: the discs were parallel to each other

and separated from each other by the atrial septum. Echo also evaluated the non-interference of the device with the surrounding structures and the absence of pericardial effusion, and excludes a significant residual shunt using color Doppler. After device release, the position of the device was again checked by echo. After the procedure, aspirin (low-dose <500 mg/day) for 6 months, transthoracic echocardiography was performed at day 1, and 1, 6, 12 months, then yearly thereafter.

Case 3 TTE-guided interventional closure via femoral vein approach in a patient with multi-fenestrated ASD (Video 4.3).

Presentation: A 45-year-old woman weighing 58 kg and with 99% SPO_2 in all limbs presented with a heart murmur that had been found during routine physical examination 1 year ago. ECG showed sinus rhythm and enlarged right atrium and ventricle. Chest X-ray showed right atrial and ventricular enlargement with increased pulmonary flow, suggesting an ASD. During a routine TTE study, the right ventricle was dilated and a small-to-moderate, left-to-right flow was observed across a fenestrated interatrial septum. The ASD was in central of atrial septum with a size of 16 mm × 10 mm, multi-fenestrated and atrial septal aneurysm. Left ventricular end diastolic diameter was 41 mm and ejection fraction was 62%.

Analysis: Patient had multi-fenestrated ASD and atrial septal aneurysm.

She should be treated by percutaneous ASD occlusion, but there might be atrial septum residual shunt after procedure, which was explained to the patient and her family. Decision was made to treat ASD by TTE-guided interventional closure via femoral vein approach using conscious sedation. If residual shunt was large or patient status was unfavorable for closure therapy, the alternative routine surgery was prepared.

Procedure: Procedure was performed in a general cardiac operating room using conscious sedation. The distance between the third intercostal space at right midclavicular line and the puncture site in right femoral vein was measured and marked on the catheter and guide wire. A sterile drape was placed between umbilical level and patient's knees. After right femoral vein puncture, arterial sheath was advanced.

The heparin 80 U/kg was administered. A 6F multipurpose catheter and a super-stiff guide wire were advanced through the sheath to ASD in the middle of atrial septum under TTE guidance. The catheter and arterial sheath then were withdrawn, and a 12F delivery sheath was advanced to left atrium along super-stiff guide wire. After guide wire and delivery sheath core withdrawal, a 26 mm ASD occluder was advanced under TTE monitoring for closure. At first, the operator deployed the device in one of the central defects, but the occluder did not cover the atrial septal aneurysm.

Delivery sheath was placed in ASD near the aortic side under TTE guidance in subsequent attempt. Then, a 28 mm occluder was deployed. Occluder location and status were appropriate. After releasing the occluder, the residual shunt disappeared. The atrial septum soft edge was covered by occluder, which did not affect the mitral valve, pulmonary vein, coronary sinus, or other surrounding cardiac structures. Compression bandages were applied after pulling out the delivery sheath and stitching the puncture site. Patient was transferred to a general ward.

Case 4 TTE-guided interventional closure via femoral vein approach in patient with ASD and atrial septum aneurysm (Video 4.4).

Presentation: A 3-year-old boy weighing 13 kg and had 100% SPO_2 in all limbs. He was diagnosed with ASD at a hospital 6 months ago and admitted to our hospital for treatment. The patient had no history of frequent colds, dyspnea on exertion, cyanosis, or syncope. ECG showed sinus rhythm. Chest X-ray: normal. Echocardiography revealed an ASD (6 mm) and atrial septum aneurysm (about 11 mm). Left ventricular end diastolic diameter was 28 mm and ejection fraction was 68%.

Analysis: The patient with an ASD (6 mm) associated with an atrial septal aneurysm, which is indication for interventional therapy. TTE-guided interventional closure via femoral vein approach was planned. Meanwhile, the preparation of routine surgery was available.

Procedure: Procedure was performed in a general cardiac operating room under general anesthesia. The distance between the third intercostal space at right midclavicular line and the puncture site in right femoral vein was measured and marked on the catheter and guide wire. A sterile drape was placed between umbilical level and patient's knees. The heparin 80 U/kg was administered. After right femoral vein puncture, a sheath was advanced.

A 6F multipurpose catheter and a super-stiff guide wire were advanced through defect under TTE guidance. The catheter and sheath then were withdrawn, and a 9F delivery sheath was advanced to left atrium along super-stiff guide wire. After guide wire and delivery sheath core withdrawal, a 15 mm ASD occluder was advanced for closure under echocardiography monitoring. Occluder location was favorable, and atrial septal aneurysm was covered by occluder. The mitral valve, pulmonary vein, coronary sinus, and surrounding structures were normal function. Compression bandages were applied after removing the delivery sheath and stitching the puncture site. The patient was transferred to general ward after consciousness.

Case 5 TEE-guided interventional closure of PFO via femoral vein approach (Video 4.5).

Presentation: A 32-year-old woman weighing 68 kg and with 100% SPO_2 in all limbs presented with migraine for 2 years without obvious inducement, cyanosis or syncope. ECG showed sinus rhythm and enlarged right atrium and ventricle. Chest X-ray showed no obvious abnormality. In TTE examination, there was no obvious abnormality of intracardiac structure at rest, while TEE examination revealed PFO. Bubble contrast echocardiography was positive.

Analysis: In this adult without obvious shunts by TTE at rest, PFO position should be confirmed to ensure the correct procedure. Therefore, TEE-guided interventional closure of PFO via femoral vein approach was planned with tracheal intubation under general anesthesia.

Procedure: The procedure was performed in a general cardiac operating room with patient under general anesthesia; tracheal intubation and echocardiography probe inserted in esophagus. PFO was about 3 mm, which met indications for percutaneous intervention. The distance between the third intercostal space at right midclavicular line and the puncture site in right femoral vein was measured and marked on the catheter and guide wire. A sterile drape was placed between umbilical level and patient's knees. After right femoral vein puncture, a sheath was introduced and heparin 80 U/kg was administered. A 6F multipurpose catheter and a super-stiff guide wire were advanced to the PFO through delivery sheath under TEE guidance. The catheter and sheath then were withdrawn, and a 10F delivery sheath was advanced to left atrium along the super-stiff guide wire. After withdrawing guide wire and delivery sheath core, an 18/25 mm PFO occluder was advanced for closure. After successful implantation, TEE parasternal short-axis view at aortic valve level and apical four-chamber view confirmed that occluder did not affect mitral valve, coronary sinus, and surrounding cardiac structures. The well-positioned and shaped occluder was released. Compression bandages were applied after pulling out the delivery sheath and stitching the puncture site. The patient was extubated in the intensive care unit and transferred to a general ward after consciousness.

Case 6 TTE-guided interventional closure of PFO via femoral vein approach (Video 4.6).

Presentation: A 48-year-old woman weighing 55 kg and with 100% SPO_2 in all limbs. She was diagnosed with PFO and had lacunar cerebral infarction 2 months ago. The patient had sudden right limb numbness 2 months ago, and the MRI suggested lacunar cerebral infarction. Bubble contrast echocardiography was positive. ECG and Chest X-ray were normal. In TTE examination, there was no obvious abnormality of heart at rest, while TEE examination revealed PFO.

Analysis: Preoperative transthoracic echocardiography examination demonstrated this patient has good echo windows. Therefore, TTE-guided interventional closure of PFO via femoral vein approach was planned with conscious sedation.

Procedure: The procedure was performed in a general cardiac operating room with patient under conscious sedation.

The patient has a history of cerebral infarction associated with PFO. She has indication for percutaneous interventional therapy. The distance between the third intercostal space at right midclavicular line and the puncture site in right femoral vein was measured and marked on the catheter and guide wire. A sterile drape was placed between umbilical level and patient's knees. After right femoral vein puncture, an arterial sheath was inserted. The heparin 80 U/kg was administered. A 6F multipurpose catheter and a super-stiff guide wire were advanced to the PFO through the arterial sheath under TTE guidance. The catheter and arterial sheath then were withdrawn, and a 10F delivery sheath was advanced to left atrium along the super-stiff guide wire. After withdrawing guide wire and delivery sheath core, a 30/30 mm PFO occluder was advanced for closure. After successful implantation, the mitral valve, aortic valve, and the surrounding structures were functioning well, which were confirmed by TTE. The well-positioned occluder was released. Compression bandages were applied after pulling out the delivery sheath and stitching the puncture site. The patient was transferred to a general ward after procedure.

References

1. Ewert P, Berger F, Daehnert I, et al. Transcatheter closure of atrial septal defects without fluoroscopy: feasibility of a new method. Circulation. 2000;101(8):847–9.
2. Zhang YSH, Zhu XY, Kong XQ, et al., Chinese expert consensus on prophylactic closure of patent foramen ovale. Chin Circ J. 2017;32(3):209–214.
3. Pan XB, Li SJ, Hu SS, et al. Feasibility of transcatheter closure of atrial septal defect under the guidance of transthoracic echocardiography. Chin J Cardiol. 2014;42(9):744–7.
4. Pan XB, Ou-Yang WB, Pang KJ, et al. Percutaneous closure of atrial septal defects under transthoracic echocardiography guidance without fluoroscopy or intubation in children. J Interv Cardiol. 2015;28(4):390–5.
5. Pan XB, Pang KJ, Hu SS, et al. Safety and efficacy of percutaneous transcatheter closure of atrial septal defect under transesophageal echocardiography guidance in children. Chin J Cardiol. 2013;41(9):744–6.

The centrally located secondary atrial septal defect (ASD) is preferably treated by interventional closure through the femoral vein approach, which does not require thoracotomy and extracorporeal circulation, and when guided by echocardiography, not only avoids conventional surgery but also avoids X-ray exposure. However, the femoral vein diameter of young patients is too small to be used as a pathway, and the jugular vein is larger than the femoral vein and can be alternative of the femoral vein. Therefore, age and weight limitations are resolved by closing the ASD through the jugular vein. This chapter introduces how to perform PAN procedure for ASD from the jugular vein.

This chapter describes techniques and methods of ASD interventional closure through jugular under echocardiography guidance.

5.1 Indications and Contraindications

1. Indications
   - Age ≥3 months, weight ≥3 kg and ≤10 kg.
   - Defect diameter ≥5 mm, at central atrial septum, with right heart volume overload.
   - The distance between the defect edge and the coronary sinus, the superior/inferior vena cava, and the pulmonary vein is ≥5 mm; the distance from the atrioventricular valve is ≥7 mm.
   - Atrial septal diameter greater than selected occluder diameter at left atrium side.
   - ASD associated with another congenital abnormality, such as inferior vena cava absence or vena cava filter placement.
   - Defects with well-defined edges except the aortic side.
2. Contraindications
   - Ostium primum or sinus venosus ASD.

Electronic Supplementary Material The online version of this chapter (https://doi.org/10.1007/978-981-15-2055-6_5) contains supplementary material, which is available to authorized users.

- Endocarditis and hemorrhagic diseases.
- There is a thrombus at the occluder location or in the vein need to insert catheter.
- Severe pulmonary hypertension with right-to-left shunt.
- Concomitant severe cardiomyopathy or valvular diseases.
- Infectious diseases within 1 month or uncontrolled infection.
- Other cardiac malformations that require surgery.
3. Patient selection

Compared to femoral vein puncture, jugular puncture is more risky and challenging due to the limited space on the head of the operating table and the sterile drape covering the patient's head and neck. Therefore, the patient must be intubated to ensure airway safety. The jugular vein pathway is only used for children with large ASD who are underweight or slow to grow and require urgent treatment. Otherwise, the femoral access is preferred regardless of the procedure guided by echocardiography or fluoroscopy. The 10–12F sheath can be inserted through the femoral vein in children weighing >10 kg.

5.2 Procedure

The procedure (Fig. 5.1) is performed in a general cardiac operating room, with patients under general anesthesia and tracheal intubation. The distance between puncture site and third intercostal space at right midclavicular line is measured and marked as working length in the catheter and guide wire. A sterile drape is placed between lips and nipples. After right jugular vein puncture, a 6F sheath is inserted. The heparin 80 U/kg is administered. A 6F multipurpose catheter (MPA2) and a super-stiff guide wire are advanced to the ASD through the sheath under echocardiography guidance. If the multipurpose catheter encounters difficulty in passing through the ASD, the pigtail catheter can be properly adjusted to guide the guide wire through the ASD. After the guide wire has

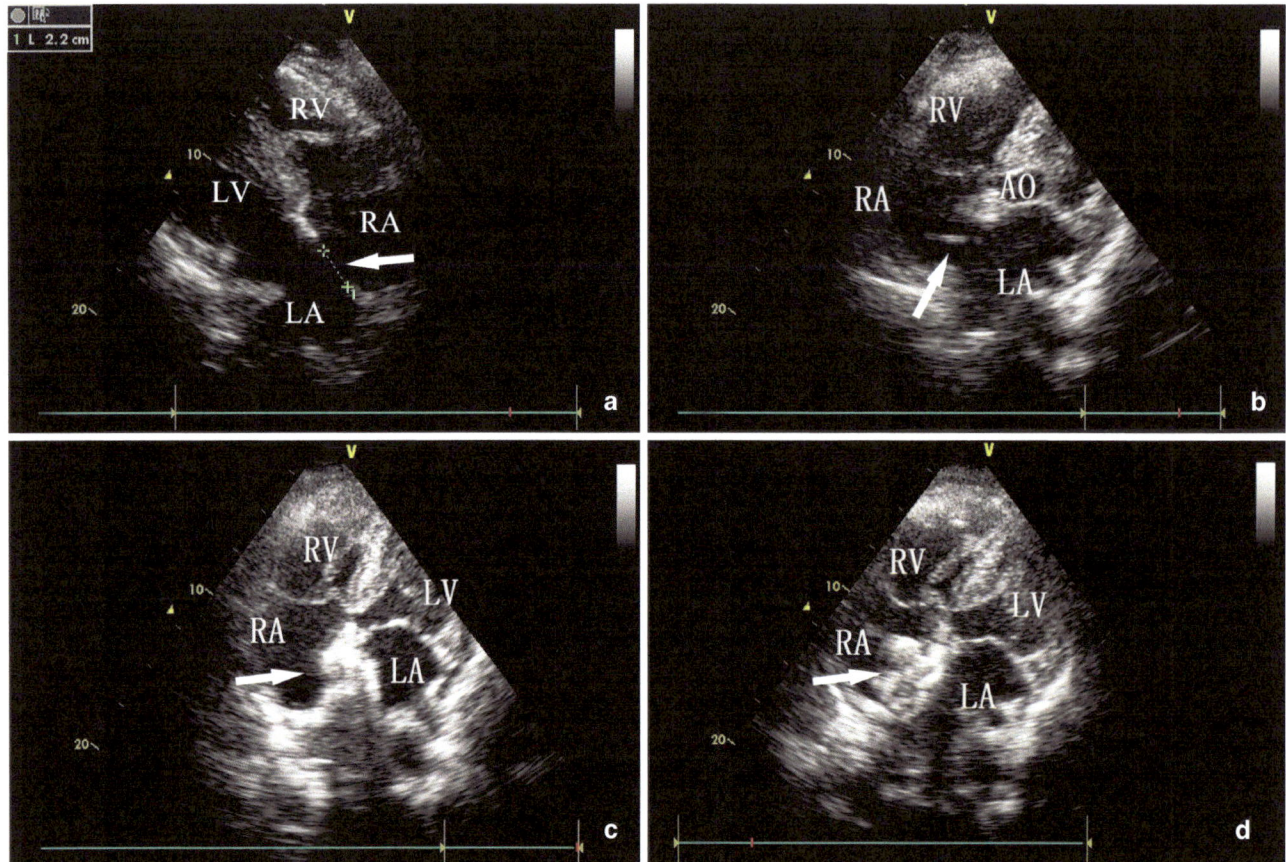

Fig. 5.1 Transthoracic echocardiography: (**a**) Parasternal four-chamber view shows the diameter of ASD (↑). (**b**) Apical four-chamber view shows the tip of catheter (↑) crossed ASD. (**c**) Apical four-chamber view shows the both sides of occluder (↑) were released. (**d**) Apical four-chamber view shows the occluder (↑) in right position. *LA* Left atrium, *RA* Right atrium, *LV* Left ventricle, *RV* Right ventricle, *AO* Aorta

passed through the ASD into the left atrium, the catheter and arterial sheath are removed. A delivery sheath with a 45° elbow is advanced along the super-stiff guide wire to the left atrium, and then the delivery sheath core is removed.

The ASD occluder then is delivered under echocardiography monitoring. Before the occluder is released, the position of occluder and the relationship with surrounding structures should be observed to confirm there is no residual shunt and the valves are functional well. The sheath was removed and then the puncture site was sutured and bandaged [1, 2].

Patients should be extubated in the operating or recovery room and then transferred to a general ward.

In some cases, a steerable sheath can be used to close the ASD through the jugular vein. The catheter's direction can be changed by control the manipulator to change the tip of steerable sheath with 0–90° flexibility. In the early stages, the steerable sheath is 100–150 cm in length and is used primarily for the aorta. Since the operating space of the neck is smaller than the space of the groin, it is inconvenient to use the long sheath through the jugular vein during the procedure. Currently, a 30–50 cm short steerable sheath is available for

jugular vein approach in clinical practice. When the sheath reaches the working length, remove the guide wire and its inner core and keep the sheath tip in the middle of the right atrium. Steer the manipulator to make the sheath curved towards the ASD. The depth and curvature of the sheath are then adjusted to deliver the occluder through the ASD under echocardiography guidance. The occluder is released after confirming the position of the occluder and not affecting the surrounding structures. The sheath is straightened by steering the manipulator and then removed. Then the puncture site is sutured and bandaged [3].

5.3   Post-procedural Treatment

After the procedure, bandage is pressed at the puncture site for 4 h while the patient remains in supine position for 12 h. Low-molecular heparin is administered subcutaneously 24 h post-procedure. Antibiotics are given intravenously once half an hour pre-procedure and 6 h post-procedure. Daily aspirin (3–5 mg/kg) is required for 6 months.

5.4 Complications Treatment

5.4.1 Occluder Malposition and Displacement, Residual Shunt, Arrhythmia and Other Complications

Refer to chapter of "Echocardiography-guided interventional ASD closure by femoral vein approach."

5.4.2 Hematoma at Puncture Site

Hematoma occurring at the puncture site occurs rarely, and hematoma occurring at the venipuncture site is mainly caused by faulty puncture and improper hemostasis. The neck tissue is slack and it is difficult to use pressurized hemostasis. The skilled anesthesiologist performs the jugular puncture with a 20-gauge trocar before procedure. The smallest sheath should be chosen. After the sheath is removed, the puncture site is recommend to be sutured and then pressurized for a sufficient period of time. In general, a small hematoma can be absorbed spontaneously without special treatment, and a large hematoma should be compressed at the puncture site, and the extravasation blood is immediately squeezed out. Indications for the use of steerable sheaths should be strictly checked. Because of the special structure of the steerable sheath, its' wall is thicker and the outer diameter of the sheath greatly exceeds the inner diameter. Thereby use of steerable sheath will increase the risk of vascular damage and hematoma, offset the advantage of the jugular vein which offers larger approach than the femoral vein.

5.4.3 Arrhythmia and Tricuspid Valve Injury

During passage through the jugular vein, the guide wire faces the tricuspid valve and the Koch's triangle after entering the right atrium. The catheter and guide wire can stimulate atrioventricular node to cause severe atrioventricular block. In addition, the risk of damage to the tricuspid chordae when using a large and rigid steerable sheath should be noted. The atrioventricular node and tricuspid valves are more easy to be damaged when adjusting the curvature of the sheath. We recommend to use the pigtail catheter to avoid damaging, because its head part is flexible and automatically bends when encountering an obstacle.

5.5 Case

Case 1 TTE-guided interventional closure of ASD by jugular vein approach in an infant (Video 5.1).

Presentation: A 1.8-year-old infant girl weighing 9 kg with 100% SPO_2 in all limbs was admitted with a heart defect found on physical examination 1 year ago. The girl suffered recurring colds, slow growth. There was no history of purpura. The electrocardiogram showed sinus rhythm; the right atrium and ventricle were enlarged. Chest X-ray examination was consistent with congenital heart disease and pulmonary blood flow increase suggesting ASD. Echocardiography showed ASD (9 mm, central), the aortic side edge was short, the distance between the defect edge and atrial posterior wall was 6 mm, and the distances from the defect edge to the superior and inferior vena cava were more than 7 mm. The left ventricular end diastolic diameter was 23 mm and the ejection fraction was 67%.

Analysis: Percutaneous closure is appropriate considering the defect size and the distances from defect edge to surrounding structures. A 15 mm occluder was chosen which required a 9F delivery sheath leading to high damage risk of transfemoral vein. Therefore, the jugular approach was adopted. Procedure: The procedure was performed in a general cardiac operating room and the patient received general anesthesia and tracheal intubation. The distance between puncture site and the third intercostal space of right midclavicular line was measured and marked on the catheter and guide wire. A sterile drape was placed in the space between the lips and the nipples. Intravenous heparin 80 U/kg was administered. A 6F sheath was inserted after the right jugular vein puncture. A 6F MPA2 catheter and guide wire were advanced through ASD under echocardiography guidance. The catheter and arterial sheath were then withdrawn, and a 9F delivery sheath was advanced along guide wire to the left atrium. After guide wire and delivery sheath core were withdrawn, a 15 mm ASD occluder was advanced under echocardiography monitoring. The occluder was released after good shape and position of the occluder, and no effect on surrounding structures were confirmed by TEE. The delivery sheath was withdrawn, the puncture site was sutured and a compression bandage was applied to the puncture site. The patient was extubated in the operating room and then transferred to the general ward when she was in stable state.

References

1. Seshagiri RD, Patnaik AN, Srinivas B. Percutaneous closure of atrial septal defect via transjugular approach with blockaid device in a patient with interrupted inferior vena cava. Cardiovasc Interv Ther. 2013;28(1):63–5.
2. Sullebarger JT, et al. Percutaneous closure of atrial septal defect via transjugular approach with the Amplatzer septal occluder after unsuccessful attempt using the CardioSEAL device. Catheter Cardiovasc Interv. 2004;62(2):262–5.
3. Xu B, Zaman S, Harper R. Successful closure of a large secundum atrial septal defect via the transjugular approach after failed transfemoral approach. Int J Cardiol. 2015;186:322–4.

Perimembranous ventricular septal defect (PmVSD) is the most common type of VSD accounting for about 70% of the total cases of VSD and typically is treated by surgery [1]. At present, percutaneous VSD closure needs to be performed under fluoroscopic guidance, with exposure to radiation. In addition, the contrast agent used for angiography may induce renal injury or allergic reaction, and the potential increased risk of complications. Echocardiography is a non-invasive imaging modality that allows assessment of valve function and measurement of blood flow velocity and pressure gradient in real time. We have practiced and proved that percutaneous VSD closure can also be performed under the guidance of echocardiography without the use of X-rays. This chapter introduces how to perform PAN procedure for VSD from femoral artery.

6.1 Anatomical Features

PmVSD is the result of maldevelopment or insufficiency of left and right heart bulbar ridges or endocardial cushion. Small PmVSD is limited to the membranous portion of the ventricular septum, while large PmVSD may affect the supraventricular crest and sinus. The superior border of the perimembranous defect is near the tricuspid valve and right coronary sinus of aorta. The atrioventricular bundle traverses the right fibrous trigone and progresses along the defect's inferior margin with both left and right branches. If the posterior defect is in the right ventricular inflow tract, the ventricular branch is close to the defect margin. When

the defect is located close to right ventricular outflow tract, ventricular bundle is further away from the defect margin. The chordae tendineae of the tricuspid valve may stretch across the defect to form two openings. The septal tricuspid valve leaflet can cover most of the defect and adhere to tissues surrounding defects contributing to ventricular septal membranous aneurysm. Therefore, during closure of PmVSD, attention should be paid to the relationship between the delivery system and the aortic valve, conducting tissues, tricuspid valve, and chordae tendineae. A suitable occluder selection may reduce the risk of conduction block and valvular regurgitation [2].

6.2 Pathophysiology

There is a close relationship between VSD pathophysiology, size and direction of shunt. After birth, left ventricular pressure is higher and pulmonary vascular resistance is reduced. The VSD provides a channel for shunting from left to right. Blood flowing into right ventricle may cause volume overload in the right heart and pulmonary circulation. Thus, intimal and medial-layer hyperplasia of the pulmonary muscular artery and arterioles may result in an increase in microvascular resistance and pulmonary hypertension. As pulmonary circulation volume increases, pulmonary vascular resistance increases and may exceed the systemic circulation resistance, the right ventricular pressure will increase and may approach or exceed the left ventricular pressure. A bidirectional or right-to-left shunt after pulmonary hypertension will result in the appearance of cyanosis and right ventricular failure as seen in patients with Eisenmenger's syndrome. For small, limited-type VSDs, i.e., patients with a defect diameter <5 mm or less than half the diameter of the aorta, the pathophysiological

Electronic Supplementary Material The online version of this chapter (https://doi.org/10.1007/978-981-15-2055-6_6) contains supplementary material, which is available to authorized users.

process is slow and does not occur in children 1–2 years of age. For large VSDs >10 mm in diameter, or close to the aortic inner diameter, the pathophysiological process can develop and this may lead to Eisenmenger's syndrome as early as few months after birth [3].

6.3 Indications and Contraindications

1. Indications
   - The patients have a simple PmVSD with abnormal hemodynamics and a defect diameter >3 mm, <10 mm.
   - The distance from superior border of VSD to the right coronary cusp of the aortic valve is ≥2 mm. The aortic right coronary valve does not prolapse into the VSD and without aortic regurgitation.
   - Age ≥2 years old and weight ≥10 kg.
2. Contraindications
   - Infective endocarditis within 6 months from intervention.
   - Severe pulmonary artery hypertension with right-to-left shunt.
   - There are other cardiac malformations that require surgery.
   - Maligned VSD.
   - Very large VSD, (diameter >10 mm).
   - The aorta overrides the edge of the VSD.
   - Aortic valve prolapse with more than mild aortic valve regurgitation.

6.4 Pre-procedural Preparation

- Explain the risks and procedures to the patient and their family and have the patient or parent sign the consent form.
- Pre-procedural examination: Routine blood and biochemical testing, coagulation function, routine physical examination, electrocardiography, and chest X-ray.
- The type and size of the VSD, the distance between the VSD and the aortic valve, whether there is a ventricular membranous aneurysm, aortic prolapse, and aortic and tricuspid regurgitation should be examined using transthoracic echocardiography.
- Prepare the skin before procedure, fasting for 8 h of solid food, and fasting of water for 6 h before procedure.

6.5 Procedure

1. The patient is in a supine position using local anesthesia or general anesthesia with spontaneous breathing. In order to ensure the safety of the patient, the puncture site of the femoral artery and the sternum area should be simultaneously sterilized for possible conventional or small chest incision surgery. Patients should receive heparin (80 U/kg). If the patient's echocardiographic image is not optimal, general anesthesia, endotracheal intubation, and jugular vein catheterization are required to guide the procedure with TEE (Fig. 6.1).

Fig. 6.1 Operating room layout

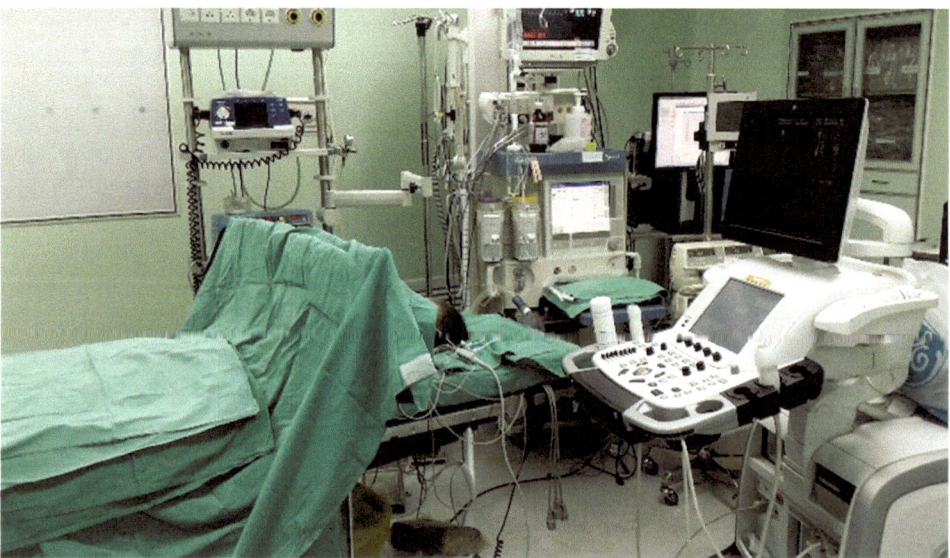

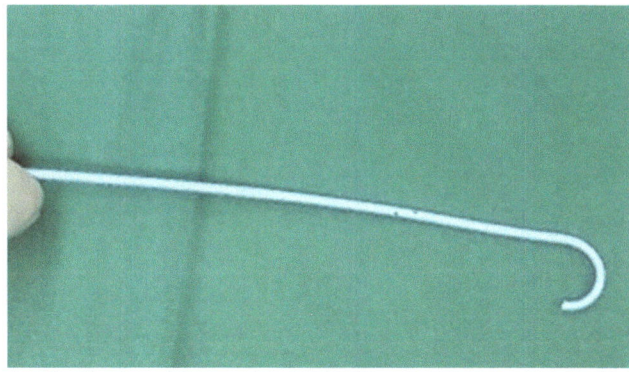

Fig. 6.2 Shape of pigtail catheter after trimming

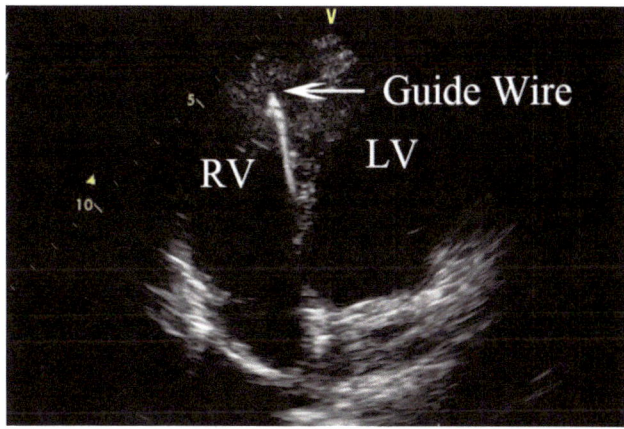

Fig. 6.4 The transthoracic echocardiography: Apical four-chamber view showing the guide wire (↑) entering the right ventricle through the VSD. *RV* Right ventricle, *LV* Left ventricle

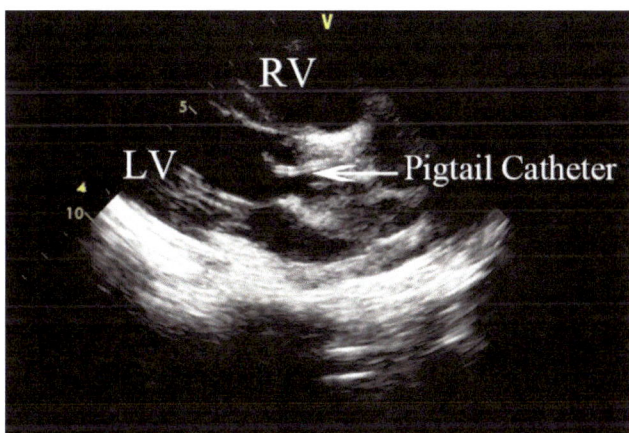

Fig. 6.3 The transthoracic echocardiography: The parasternal long-axis view shows that trimmed pigtail catheter (↑) is in left ventricular outflow tract and its top faces the defect. *RV* Right ventricle, *LV* Left ventricle

Gently push the catheter along the guide wire into the ascending aorta and withdraw the guide wire. Guided by a parasternal long-axis view showing the long axis of the ascending aorta, the catheter is rotated and gently advanced through the aortic valve to the left ventricle, to avoid damaging the aortic valve.

5. After the catheter enters the left ventricle, adjust the direction of the pigtail catheter so that its top faces the defect (Fig. 6.3). Using the long-axis view of the aorta or the five-chamber view as a guide, the guide wire is gently advanced into the right ventricle through the VSD. This process is a key step. If resistance is encountered during guide wire push, indicating that the guide wire is striking the ventricular septum, the orientation of guide wire should be adjusted under echocardiography guidance. Sometimes, if the image is not ideal, it is difficult to determine if the guide wire has entered the right ventricle through the VSD. The location of the guide wire should be verified in a four-chamber view (Fig. 6.4).

6. Prior to procedure, the occluder selected should be 1–2 mm larger than the diameter of the defect measured by echocardiography.

7. The pigtail catheter is withdrawn and the depth of insertion is marked as working length. The delivery sheath is advanced along the guide wire to a depth 2–4 cm deeper than the depth of insertion of the pigtail catheter, and the catheter enters the right ventricle through the VSD verified by echocardiographic guidance. The delivery sheath dilator and guide wire are removed and the occluder is advanced along the delivery sheath and right-side disc is deployed in the right ventricle. The delivery system is then withdrawn to place the right-side disc of occluder close to

2. The distance between the second left intercostal space and the puncture site in right femoral artery is measured as working length. Puncture the right femoral artery and insert a 5F arterial sheath. According to the echocardiographic parasternal long-axis view, the direction of the VSD shunt is shown, and trim the tip of the 5F pigtail catheter to form a 1/3–1/2 curved bend (Fig. 6.2).

3. The 5F pigtail catheter and guide wire (the tip of which can extend 2–3 cm from the catheter) are delivered as a unit through the arterial sheath. After the catheter enters the artery from the femoral artery puncture site, it should be gently advanced under echocardiography guidance.

4. When the catheter and guide wire reach the working length, the guide wire and the pigtail catheter enter the ascending aorta under the guidance of the aortic arch view from the suprasternal notch window, and the pigtail catheter is adjusted to the lesser curvature of the aortic arch.

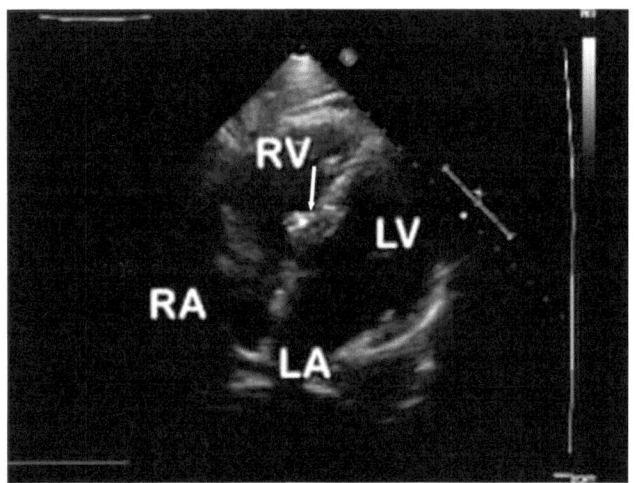

Fig. 6.5 The occluder's right disc (↑) is deployed in the right ventricle, and the delivery system is pulled back to make the right disc close to the right side of defect

the defect (Fig. 6.5). If resistance is encountered during pulling back to the ventricular septum, the occluder maybe entangled by the tricuspid valve chordae. The occluder should be withdrawn into the sheath slightly. Make the tip of sheath just passed the defect into the right ventricle. The occluder's right-side disc is then deployed again in the right ventricle, and after this disc covering the right side of the defect is confirmed, the delivery sheath is withdrawn to deploy the left-side disc of the occluder to cover the left side of the defect.

8. The position of the occluder and its relationship to the aortic valve should be evaluated in the parasternal long-axis or apical 4-chamber view. Doppler echocardiography is performed to examine residual shunt and new tricuspid regurgitation or exacerbation of the regurgitation. Aortic valve regurgitation may result from the delivery catheter passing through the aortic valve prior to release of the occluder. Two-dimensional echocardiography is used to observe whether the aortic valve leaflet was compressed by the occluder. If there is no compression, the aortic valve regurgitation will disappear after the occluder is released.

9. If the occluder is properly positioned, rotate the delivery catheter counterclockwise to release the occluder, and remove the delivery system. The shape and position of the occluder and the function of the aortic valve are assessed again by echocardiography. The puncture site is badged and compressed to achieve hemostasis [4–6].

6.6 Postoperative Treatment

1. The puncture site is manually pressed for few minutes until hemostasis is achieved and the patient is asked to lay flat on his/her back for 6 h. The patient is observed in the hospital for 24 h. A sedative can be used as appropriate.

2. Low-molecular heparin is administered subcutaneously 24 h post-procedure.

3. Since the first day after procedure, aspirin (3–5 mg/kg) is orally administered for 6 months.

4. Echocardiography, ECG, and chest X-ray are performed within 24 h after procedure.

5. Antibiotics are given intravenously once half an hour pre-procedure and 6 h post-procedure.

6. Echocardiography and electrocardiography should be performed at 1 month, 3 months, and 6 months after procedure.

6.7 Complications

6.7.1 Occluder Displacement or Embolization

Occluder displacement or embolization is a rare complication. Occluder may migrate to left ventricle, aorta, right ventricle, or pulmonary artery. The occluder can be percutaneously retrieved by Amplatz goose neck snare or surgically removed. Proper sedation should be given early in the postoperative period and intense activity should be strictly prohibited within 6 months after procedure.

6.7.2 Peripheral Vascular Injury

Echocardiography-guided percutaneous VSD closure via femoral artery avoids femoral vein injury. Femoral artery puncture should be performed using the modified Seldinger technique. The process or pathway of guide wire and catheter advanced into the ascending aorta from the femoral artery are unvisible by echocardiographic monitoring. The operator should handle this carefully. If resistance is encountered, the guide wire and catheter should be withdrawn slightly to try again.

6.7.3 Tricuspid Regurgitation

Echocardiography-guided transfemoral ventricular septal defect occlusion does not require an arteriovenous loop, thus reducing the risk of damage to the tricuspid valve and its chordae. If resistance is encountered during the deployment of right disc, the occluder may be caught by the tricuspid chordae. The sheath should be pulled back slightly to make the tip of sheath just passed the defect into the right ventricle. The right disc of the occluder is then deployed again in the right ventricle. If tricuspid regurgitation occurs or the original tricuspid regurgitation is aggravated, the deployment procedure should be repeated.

6.7.4 Aortic Valve Regurgitation

The most important method to prevent aortic regurgitation is to select the patient before procedure; the distance between the defect edge and the aortic valve should be >2 mm. In addition, it is important to carefully evaluate the position of aortic valve and the left-side disc of the occluder before releasing the occluder.

6.7.5 Atrioventricular Block

The tissue surrounding the PmVSD compressed by the occluder can lead to inflammation and edema, which most often cause the right bundle branch block, or complete atrioventricular block as the most serious complication. The incidence of conduction block is reported to be 0–22%, and risk factors for AV block caused by ventricular septal defect closure include low body weight and large occlude size. It is recommended to use an occluder that is 1–2 mm larger than the defect and use a new modified occluder with increased waist length, or other new occluder (Nit-Occlud® LêVSD occluder, Amplatzer2 Membrane VSD occluder) can reduce the incidence of AV block. Since it is unnecessary to establish a loop, thus the risks of compressing or stimulating the surrounding tissue of the defect and subsequent postoperative atrioventricular block are decreased signicantly.

6.7.6 Residual Shunt

According to Yang et al.'s literature review, residual shunt is the most common complication after VSD closure [4]. Of the 4138 patients who underwent percutaneous VSD closure in 35 studies, 1134 patients (27.4%) had postoperative residual shunt. A trivial residual shunt can spontaneously disappear after the procedure. According to our experience, if the width of the residual shunt is >2 mm, transthoracic closure or surgery should be performed.

6.7.7 Air Embolism

Care should be taken to manipulate the catheter and exchange the guide wire. When the occluder reaches the end of the delivery sheath but has not yet been deployed, the blood is withdrawn with a syringe to fill the delivery sheath with blood, thereby reducing the risk of air embolism.

6.7.8 Hemolysis

It has been reported that the incidence of hemolysis is 0.7–15% after VSD closure, and hemolysis mainly occurs in the early postoperative period, especially in patients with residual shunt. Most patients can receive glucocorticoid therapy, otherwise surgery should be performed to remove the occluder and repair the VSD. The routine blood, urine, and free hemoglobin should be tested for all patients with residual shunt.

6.7.9 Pericardial Effusion

Pericardial effusion rarely occurs after percutaneous closure, which may be caused by the catheter and guide wire piercing the myocardium during procedure. Careful and gentle manipulation is very important.

6.8 Summary

There are only a few reports of echocardiography-guided VSD closure via femoral artery; Fuwai Hospital first reported patients who were treated between February 2014 and March 2015. This report included 42 patients with PmVSD who underwent echocardiography-guided VSD closure. The procedures were successfully completed in 36 patients. The catheter was failed to cross the VSD in 2 patients. Instead, echocardiography-guided transthoracic closure through a small chest incision was performed. The other 2 patients underwent routine surgery for residual shunt >2 mm. Four patients had a trivial residual shunt immediately after procedure and disappeared after 1 month. Right bundle branch block occurred in 3 patients, 2 of them recovered before discharge. After 6 months of follow-up, all patients had no complications such as pericardial effusion, occluder displacement, atrioventricular block, or hemolysis. Peripheral VSD closure through femoral artery guided by echocardiography solely is as safe and effective as by fluoroscopy, while avoiding exposure to radiation and contrast agents and excluding the establishment of the arteriovenous loop. Therefore, it has obvious advantages in preventing related valve damage. This technique is difficult to master and requires a long learning curve. Therefore, teams using this technology should be trained to achieve the proficiency of the required technical skills and set strict guidelines. This technology has the great potential to be widely developed and applied.

6.9 Cases

Case 1 A 5.6-year-old boy, weight 17 kg (Video 6.1).

The patient was admitted to hospital with heart murmur detected 10 months prior to the procedure. There was no history of cyanosis after crying and screaming. However, he was susceptible to colds, and his weight was lower than children of the same age, with no history of hemoptysis or syncope.

On physical examination, a grade 3 rough pan systolic murmur was heard between the left third and fourth intercostal space. Chest X-ray showed both left and right lungs congestion. The electrocardiogram showed high voltage of the left ventricle. Echocardiography showed a PmVSD, diameter 3.5 mm, and 3 mm distance to the aortic valve and mild regurgitation of the tricuspid valve. TTE-guided PmVSD closure was performed by the femoral artery approach. The patient was in the supine position and given a sedative. This procedure was performed under the guidance of TTE. The 6F sheath was inserted into the right femoral artery. The 5F pigtail catheter was trimmed and used to guide the guide wire through the VSD. After removal of the pigtail catheter, the 5F delivery sheath was delivered through the ventricular septal defect and a 6 mm ventricular septal defect occluder was deployed and the closure was successful. There were no complications after procedure, including residual shunt, conduction block, pericardial effusion, and hemolysis.

Case 2 32-year-old man, weight 89 kg (Video 6.2).

The patient was admitted with a heart murmur detected 6 years ago. He was susceptible to colds, and fatigue, but no history of hemoptysis or syncope. On physical examination, a grade 3 rough pan systolic murmur was heard between the left third and fourth intercostal space. Chest X-ray showed both of left and right lungs congestion. The electrocardiogram showed incomplete right bundle branch block. Echocardiography showed a 5 mm PmVSD with 4 mm distance to the aortic valve.

TTE image quality was not good enough for guidance. TEE-guided PmVSD closure was performed by the femoral artery approach. The patient was given general anesthesia with tracheal intubation and echo probe in esophagus. Under TEE guidance, a 6F sheath was inserted after puncturing the right femoral artery. A 5F pigtail catheter was trimmed and used to guide guide wire through VSD. After withdrawing the pigtail catheter, a 5F delivery sheath with a 7 mm VSD occluder was advanced through VSD for closure. There were no post procedural complications, i.e., residual shunt, conduction block, pericardial effusion, and hemolysis.

References

1. Butera G, et al. Transcatheter closure of perimembranous ventricular septal defects: early and long-term results. J Am Coll Cardiol. 2007;50(12):1189–95.
2. Carminati M, et al. Transcatheter closure of congenital ventricular septal defects: results of the European registry. Eur Heart J. 2007;28(19):2361–8.
3. Fu YC, et al. Transcatheter closure of perimembranous ventricular septal defects using the new Amplatzer membranous VSD occluder: results of the U.S. phase I trial. J Am Coll Cardiol. 2006;47(2):319–25.
4. Pan XB, Pang KJ, Ouyang WB, et al. Application of percutaneous ventricular septal defect closure under solely guidance of echocardiography. Chin Circ J. 2015;30(8):774–6.
5. Tzikas A, et al. Transcatheter closure of perimembranous ventricular septal defect with the Amplatzer((R)) membranous VSD occluder 2: initial world experience and one-year follow-up. Catheter Cardiovasc Interv. 2014;83(4):571–80.
6. Yang J, et al. Transcatheter device closure of perimembranous ventricular septal defects: mid-term outcomes. Eur Heart J. 2010;31(18):2238–45.

7.1 Anatomical Features

PmVSD is the result of maldevelopment or insufficiency of left and right heart bulbar ridges or endocardial cushion. Small PmVSD is limited to the membranous portion of the ventricular septum, while large PmVSD may affect the supraventricular crest and sinus. The superior border of the perimembranous defect is near the tricuspid valve and right coronary sinus of aorta. The atrioventricular bundle traverses the right fibrous trigone and progresses along the defect's inferior margin with both left and right branches. If the posterior defect is in the right ventricular inflow tract, the ventricular branch is close to the defect margin. When the defect is located close to right ventricular outflow tract, ventricular bundle is further away from the defect margin. The chordae tendineae of the tricuspid valve may stretch across the defect to form two openings. The septal tricuspid valve leaflet can cover most of the defect and adhere to tissues surrounding defects contributing to ventricular septal membranous aneurysm. Therefore, during closure of PmVSD, attention should be paid to the relationship between the delivery system and the aortic valve, conducting tissues, tricuspid valve, and chordae tendineae. A suitable occluder selection may reduce the risk of conduction block and valvular regurgitation.

7.2 Pathophysiology

There is a close relationship between VSD pathophysiology, size and direction of shunt. After birth, left ventricular pressure is higher and pulmonary vascular resistance is reduced. The VSD provides a channel for shunting from left to right. Blood flowing into right ventricle may cause volume overload in the

right heart and pulmonary circulation. Thus, intimal and medial-layer hyperplasia of the pulmonary muscular artery and arterioles may result in an increase in microvascular resistance and pulmonary hypertension. As pulmonary circulation volume increases, pulmonary vascular resistance increases and may exceed the systemic circulation resistance, the right ventricular pressure will increase and may approach or exceed the left ventricular pressure. A bidirectional or right-to-left shunt after pulmonary hypertension will result in the appearance of cyanosis and right ventricular failure as seen in patients with Eisenmenger's syndrome. For small, limited-type VSDs, i.e., patients with a defect diameter <5 mm or less than half the diameter of the aorta, the pathophysiological process is slow and does not occur in children 1–2 years of age. For large VSDs >10 mm in diameter, or close to the aortic inner diameter, the pathophysiological process can develop and this may lead to Eisenmenger's syndrome as early as few months after birth.

7.3 Indications and Contraindications

1. Indications
   - Weight ≥5 kg.
   - Perimembranous VSD, abnormal hemodynamics, diameter >3 to <10 mm.
   - The distance between the upper edge of VSD and the right coronary cups of the aortic valve is ≥2 mm, there is no aortic right coronary valve prolapse, or aortic valve regurgitation.
   - Infracristal VSD near the aortic valve. If the defect diameter is <5 mm and the distance from the pulmonary valve is >2 mm, most of patients may successfully close the defect; however, long-term efficacy remains to be seen. A typical VSD can be closed via the jugular vein, especially in infants with a light weight, because the jugular vein has a relatively large diameter and is more accessible than the femoral vein.

Electronic Supplementary Material The online version of this chapter (https://doi.org/10.1007/978-981-15-2055-6_7) contains supplementary material, which is available to authorized users.

In addition, the VSD at the posterior part of the ventricular septum should be prefered to be closed via the jugular vein to reduce the curvature of the delivery sheath and avoid the resistance during passing through septum defect.

2. Contraindications
   • Infective endocarditis or other infectious diseases.
   • There is a thrombus in the place where the occluder will be placed.
   • Very large VSD and poor anatomic location of defect. After placement, occluder may affect the function of aortic or atrioventricular valve.
   • Severe pulmonary artery hypertension with right-to-left shunt.
   • Second- or third-degree atrioventricular block.
   • Hemorrhagic diseases and thrombocytopenia.
   • Abnormal hepatic-renal function.
   • Heart failure and intolerance to procedure.
   • Concomitant with other cardiac malformations that require surgery.

7.4   Pre-procedural Evaluation

Physical examination and transthoracic echocardiography, chest X-ray, electrocardiogram, routine blood test, liver and kidney function, electrolyte, coagulation function, and infectious disease indicators should be performed.

In transthoracic echocardiography, the location, size and shape of the VSD, and the distance between the defect edge and the aortic valve were evaluated to assess the relationship between the VSD and the Koch triangle apex. For patients with membranous septum aneurysm, the diameter, number, and size of defect in basilar part of septum should be determined (Fig. 7.1a). The VSD size and distance between defect margin and aortic valve should be measured in parasternal or apical five-chamber views. In order to guide the entry of the guide wire, the location, size, and direction of the defect should be observed in the aortic level of parasternal short-axis view. The relationship between the defect and the aortic valve and the presence of aortic valve prolapse can be observed in the parasternal long-axis view. The relationship

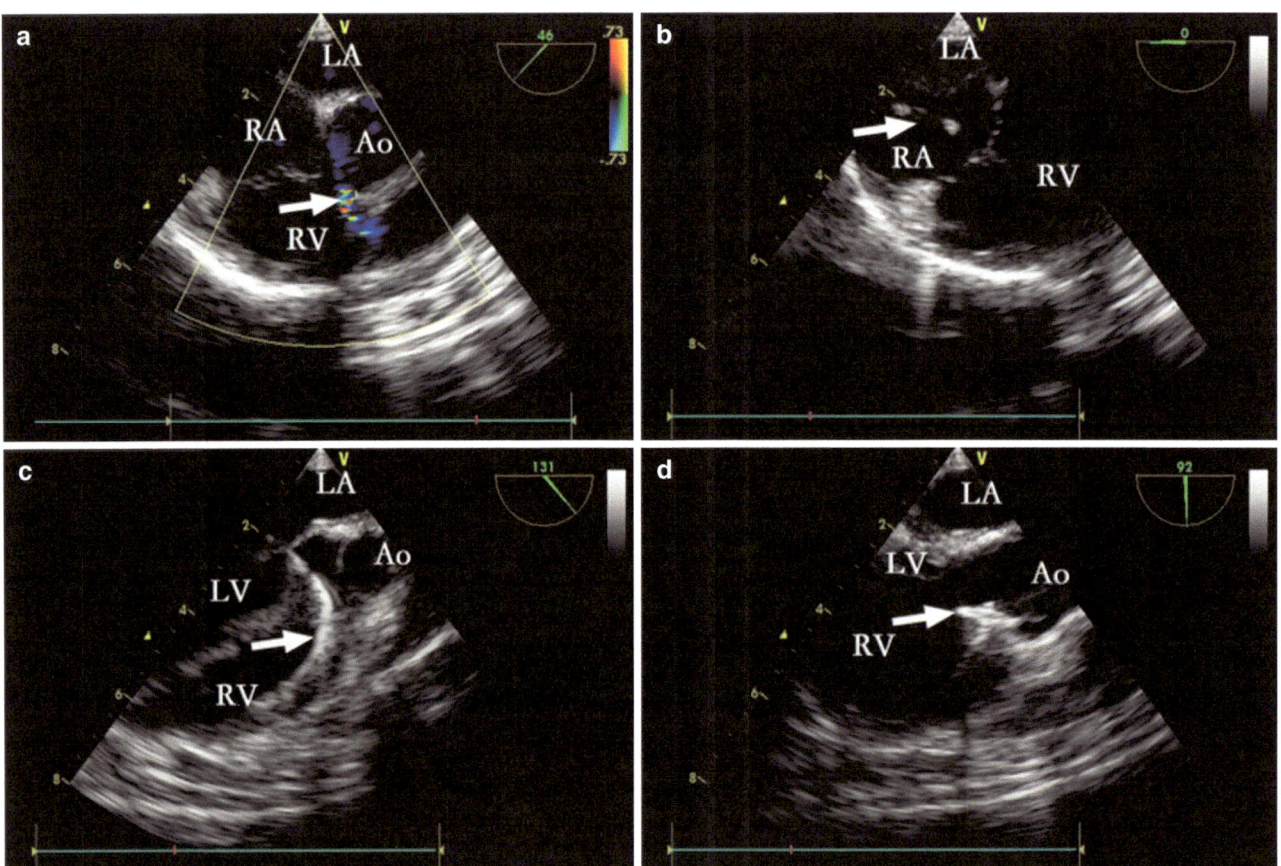

Fig. 7.1 TEE echocardiography in VSD closure by jugular vein approach. (**a**) The left to right shunt (↑) through VSD. (**b**) The distal end of catheter (↑) is in right atrium. (**c**) Guide wire (↑) crosses VSD into left ventricle. (**d**) The left disc of occluder (↑) is deployed. *AO* Ascending aorta, *LA* Left atrium, *LV* Left ventricle, *RA* Right atrium, *RV* Right ventricle

between the tricuspid valve and the VSD can be seen in the aortic level of the parasternal short-axis view and in the apical or parasternal five-chamber views [1].

7.5 Procedure

Patients should be in supine position with tracheal intubation under general anesthesia and TEE probe should be inserted. Some adult patients could undergo the procedure with local anesthesia, and sedative, without tracheal intubation, and guided by transthoracic echocardiography. It should be emphasized that when the jugular vein is inserted, the operating area is located at the head of the operating table, and the patient's face is covered with a sterile drape, making it difficult for the anesthesiologist to observe and ensure the airway is unobstructed. In addition, patients may be afraid and anxious, so most of patients should receive general anesthesia with endotracheal intubation. After sterilizing the skin and puncturing the right jugular vein, the distance between the puncture site and the right third intercostal space is measured and labeled as working length to determine the depth of insertion of the delivery system into the body.

After establishing access, heparin 80–100 U/kg is regularly administered. A 5F arterial sheath is introduced via the jugular vein. Because of young age and low weight of patients, while the expander of 5F arterial sheath is long, the expander should be pulled out gradually while inserting the arterial sheath into vessel to avoid heart damage. Moreover, the arterial sheath should not be completely inserted to avoid injuring intracardiac structure such as tricuspid valve. Insertion depth of the arterial sheath should be 3–5 cm, and the arterial sheath should be fixed to sterile towel by stitches. Trim the 5F pigtail catheter according to the VSD direction so that its proximal end is bent in 1/2–3/4 arc. The pigtail catheter and guide wire are delivered through the arterial sheath to working length. The guide wire is then withdrawn and the catheter rotated under echocardiographic guidance to detect its location and direction (Fig. 7.1b). After catheter direction is adjusted, it is advanced to right ventricle through tricuspid valve and then catheter direction is readjusted with its top facing the VSD. Guided by the aortic level of the parasternal short-axis view, the guide wire is gently pushed to determine its position and adjusted to deliver the guide wire to the left ventricle via the VSD (Fig. 7.1c).

In some patients, after repeated adjustment of the catheter direction, the guide wire is still difficult to pass the ventricular septal defect. Under this circumstance, a 5F steerable catheter can be used. The distal end of catheter curvature can be adjusted in 0–90° range, allowing delivering catheter to right atrium through jugular vein in a straight line. Using the manipulator, the proximal end of the catheter is rotated to gradually bend to the proper curvature, allowing the catheter to easily pass through the VSD (Fig. 7.2). However, the steerable catheter is thicker (the outer diameter is 2F larger than the inner diameter), may damage the tricuspid chordae, thus preserving as an alternative to conventional methods.

After the guide wire enters in the left ventricle through the ventricular septum, the catheter is withdrawn and the guide wire is retained for guiding the delivery sheath. When the catheter is withdrawn, its insertion length should be measured as a reference for the insertion of the delivery sheath. Because the left ventricle of young children is small, the guide wire enters the left ventricle at a smaller depth and cannot provide sufficient support. For this type of patient, the snare can be placed through the femoral artery into the ascending aorta and opened to adjust the direction of the guide wire. Thus, the guide wire passes the VSD and the aortic valve into the ascending aorta. The guide wire is captured using a snare to establish a jugular vein-VSD-femoral artery circuit. You can transfer the delivery catheter along the guide wire into the jugular vein-ventricular septum-femoral artery path to close the VSD.

The selection of occluder. In the preoperative echocardiography, the diameter of the VSD should be measured, and an occluder which is 1–3 mm larger than the diameter of the VSD should be selected. For patients with VSD away from the aortic valve, a symmetric occluder is preferred. If the VSD is close to the aortic valve, an asymmetrical occluder should be chosen. For multifenestrated defects, a thin waist occluder with asymmetric size disc should be selected.

Under echocardiographic monitoring, the delivery sheath is advanced along the guide wire and passed through the VSD into the left ventricle. The delivery sheath core and guide wire are removed and the occluder is advanced through the delivery sheath into the left ventricle, deployed the left disc of the occluder (Fig. 7.1d). Withdraw the delivery system to bring the occluder close to the VSD. The right disc of the occluder is then deployed. If an eccentric occluder is used, after the left disc is deployed, under the aortic long-axis view, rotate the occluder to make the marker in left disc away from the aortic valve.

Echocardiography can be used to assess residual shunt, whether the occluder is remote from the aortic valve, and whether there is aortic regurgitation. After repeated push-pull tests, it was confirmed that there was no displacement, residual shunt, or valve regurgitation, the heart rhythm was normal, and then the delivery catheter was rotated counterclockwise to release the occluder [2–4].

The delivery system is removed and the puncture site is bandaged and compressed to control bleeding.

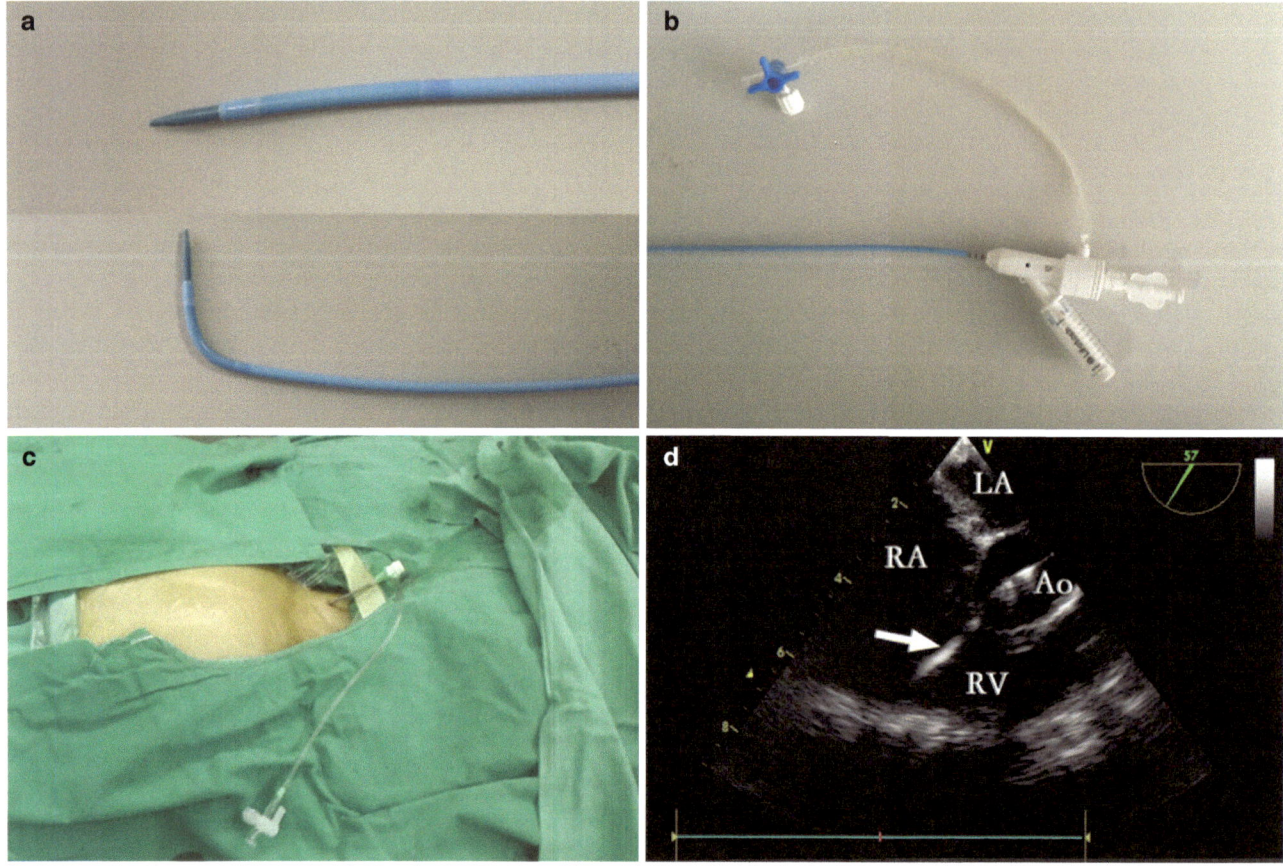

Fig. 7.2 Steerable catheter. (**a**) The distal end of steerable catheter can be adjusted in 0–90° range. (**b**) The proximal end of steerable catheter. (**c**) Operating sheath in right jugular vein. (**d**) Guide wire of steerable catheter (↑) is crossing VSD. *AO* Ascending aorta, *LA* Left atrium, *LV* Left ventricle, *RA* Right atrium, *RV* Right ventricle

7.6   Post-procedural Treatment

- Patients should be monitored. The electrocardiogram, TTE, and chest X-ray should be performed within 24 h of procedure.
- Low-molecular heparin is administered subcutaneously 24 h post-procedure. Antibiotics are given intravenously once half an hour pre-procedure and 6 h post-procedure.
- Aspirin orally: infants, 3–5 mg/(kg·day); and adults, 100–200 mg/day for 6 months.
- Intensive exercise should be avoided within 6 months after procedure. The patients should be followed up, and the TTE and ECG should be performed at 1, 3, 6, and 12 months after procedure. Chest X-ray should be obtained if necessary.

7.7   Complications and Treatment

7.7.1   Occluder Displacement

The occluder displacement may occur because the occluder is too small or the operation is improper. The occluder can migrate to the left ventricle, aorta, right ventricle, or pulmonary artery. If the occluder migrates, it can be trapped and taken out by a snare, the long sheath should be as close as possible to the occluder to reduce the risk of critical heart structural injuries. If the occluder cannot be taken out, or if hemodynamic changes are caused by occluder migration, the occluder should be removed by surgery under extracorporeal circulation and the VSD should be repaired simutaneously.

7.7.2   Arrhythmia

Although ventricular premature beats, ventricular tachycardia, bundle branch block, and atrioventricular block may occur during the procedure, most of them may disappear after adjusting the guide wire and catheter. Accelerated idioventricular rhythm occurs primarily in patients with VSD close to right ventricular outflow tract or the perimambraneous VSD extends to adjacent muscular septum. It is caused by the stimulation from the occluder during the procedure. If ventricular rate is <100/min, no medication is needed. Ventricular fibrillation is rare but can occur when the catheter or guide wire strongly stimulates the ventricular myocardium.

Hypokalemia should be avoided before procedure. Once ventricular fibrillation occurs, electrical cardioversion should be performed immediately. Third-degree atrioventricular block and junctional escape rhythm are associated with occluder size, VSD type, and procedural injury. If the junctional escapes rhythm occurs with a third degree of atrioventricular block, and the heart rate is >55 beats/min and the QRS interval is within 0.12 s, dexamethasone can be administered intravenously (child: 0.2 mg/kg/day; adult: 10 mg/day) for 3–7 days. Under close observation, if the ventricular rate is too slow or Adams–Stokes syndrome occurs, a temporary cardiac pacemaker should be implanted. If the patient does not recover after 3 weeks, a permanent pacemaker should be implanted or transfer to surgical operation. Third-degree atrioventricular block mainly occurs early in the postoperative period, although there is evidence in recent years that it may occur in advanced stages, so long-term follow-up is needed.

7.7.3 Chordae Tendinous Rupture

Since the guide wire must pass through the gap between the chordae tendineae to establish a path, the chordae may be damaged. Typically, rupture of the mitral chordae is caused by forced manipulation of the delivery sheath into the left ventricle, particularly when the delivery catheter of occluder is advancing or withdrawing. Since the hardness of the adjustable curved catheter is much larger than that of the pigtail catheter, it should be carefully rotated after entering the right ventricle, otherwise the chordae tendinous injury may occur once the catheter is entangled with the tricuspid chordae. This procedure should be performed with care and gentleness, especially in babies. Once the chordae rupture occurs, the chordae and ventricular septal defect should be repaired by surgery immediately under cardiopulmonary bypass.

7.7.4 Tricuspid Regurgitation

It is related to the defect location, the operation mode, and the size of the occluder. The defect is closer to the tricuspid valve, and the insertion of the occluder can cause significant tricuspid regurgitation. When releasing the occluder, the push rod should be rotated while pushing the distal end of the sheath close to the occluder to prevent entanglement with the chordae. Too large occluder, the waist of the occluder is limited due to the small defect, and the edge expends relatively long, or the occluder disc forms a spherical appearance, which occupies a large space after release, may lead to tricuspid regurgitation. If an obvious tricuspid regurgitation is found during the procedure, the closure process should be abandoned.

7.7.5 Aortic Valve Regurgitation

The risk of aortic regurgitation is associated with occluder and operation. If the edge of the left disc is larger than the distance between the VSD and the aortic valve, occluder may affect the function of the aortic valve. Once the aortic regurgitation develops, the VSD repairing and occluder removing should be performed by surgery under extracorporeal circulation.

7.7.6 Residual Shunt

Significant residual shunts occur mainly in patients with porous VSD, often because the occluder does not completely cover the defect surface. The left disc should cover the defect completely. Generally, for residual shunts <2 mm or a transseptum velocity <3 m/s, no special treatment is required and may disappear in a short period after procedure. If the residual shunt is still >2 mm or its velocity > 3 m/s at 6 months after procedure, the occluder removal and the ventricular septal defect repairing should be performed by surgery.

7.7.7 Hemolysis

It is related to the existence of residual shunt. A high-velocity blood flow through the occluder can cause hemolysis, manifested as dark urine, chills, anemia, renal insufficiency, etc., which should be closely observed. For mild hemolysis, aspirin should be discontinued, intravenous hemostasis and oral or intravenous sodium bicarbonate should be given. If the hemoglobin is <70 g/L, the occluder should be removed by surgery under extracorporeal circulation.

7.7.8 Air Embolism

The catheter and guide wire should be manipulated carefully to reduce risk of air embolism.

7.7.9 Acute Myocardial Infarction

In China, there have been few reports of acute extensive anterior myocardial infarction after intervention, which may be due to intra-catheter thrombosis falling into the coronary artery due to insufficient anticoagulation during the intervention procedure. Such complications are rare and can be difficult to deal with. Intraoperative anticoagulation should be performed, usually heparin is given at 80–100 U/kg, or heparin dose is administered according to ACT monitoring results. After procedure, close observation is needed and ECG should be given in time if patients had symptoms such as abdominal pain or chest pain. Thrombolytic therapy is feasible by early dignosis.

7.7.10 Heart and Vessel Perforation

Mostly, it is caused by rough operation when advancing the delivery sheath. Therefore, the operation must be gentle. After the end of the closure, pericardial effusion should be carefully examined. If there is perforation and rupture, it should be repaired by surgery immediately.

7.8   Case

Case A 6-year-old boy, weighing 16.5 kg (Video 7.1).

The patient was admitted for a heart murmur found more than 4 years ago. Patient was poor in growth and susceptible to colds. A 3/6 pan systolic murmur could be heard between third and fourth intercostal spaces at the left sternal border. Echocardiographic findings: perimembranous ventricular septal defect, diameter was 4.4 mm, the edge of the defect was about 3 mm distance to the aortic valve. The electrocardiogram showed sinus rhythm and left ventricular high voltage. Chest X-ray showed congestion in both of left and right lungs. VSD closure was performed through the jugular vein under general anesthesia. The right jugular vein was punctured and the 6F arterial sheath was inserted. The guide wire and catheter were advanced through the arterial sheath. After the catheter passed through the VSD, the 5F delivery sheath was advanced. A 7 mm VSD occluder was delivered through the delivery sheath and deployed. Low-molecular heparin was administered subcutaneously 24 h post-procedure, 50 mg/day oral aspirin was prescribed for 6 months, and antibiotics are given intravenously once half an hour pre-procedure and 6 h post-procedure. Echocardiography, electrocardiography, and chest radiography showed no abnormality, and the patient was discharged on the third day.

References

1. Zhou T, et al. Percutaneous closure of ventricular septal defect associated with anomalous inferior vein cava drainage via transjugular approach. Chin Med J (Engl). 2005;118(7):615–6.
2. Lee SM, et al. Transcatheter closure of perimembranous ventricular septal defect using Amplatzer ductal occluder. Catheter Cardiovasc Interv. 2013;82(7):1141–6.
3. Pan XB, Ou-Yang WB, Wang SZ, et al. Exploration research of ventricular septal defect closure via trans-jugular approach solely under the guidance of echocardiography. Chin Circ J. 2016;30(12):1204–7.
4. Yang L, et al. A systematic review on the efficacy and safety of transcatheter device closure of ventricular septal defects (VSD). J Interv Cardiol. 2014;27(3):260–72.

Patent ductus arteriosus (PDA) is one of the common congenital heart diseases, accounting for 7–10% of cases and ranking third among all the heart diseases. The arterial duct, as part of the fetal circulation, is an important blood channel between the pulmonary artery and aorta during the fetal stage. The fetus does not breathe without an independent pulmonary circulation, mainly depending on the arterial duct for oxygenated blood supply. After birth, with the establishment of spontaneous breathing, independent pulmonary circulation, reduction in pulmonary vascular resistance and pulmonary circulation pressure, the arterial duct of most infants will automatically close within 1 year and degenerate into an arterial ligament. Otherwise, a PDA persists. This chapter introduces how to perform PAN procedure for PDA from femoral artery.

The yearly increase in mortality of patients with hemodynamic changes associated with PDA is 0.49% in the 2–19 years old and reaches 1.8% in the >20 years old, respectively, 30% of them died of congestive heart failure. Therefore, infants with PDA featuring significant hemodynamic changes should be treated proactively with surgery or interventions. In 1966, Porstmann first successfully occluded the arterial duct with an Ivalon plug [1], the surgical operation, and the interventional therapy co-existing for PDA at that time. Thereafter, different occluders including Rashkind Double-Umbrella occlusion device, occluding spring coils, and Amplatzer mushroom-shaped devices, etc., have been used for the PDA treatment. The Spring Bolt by COOK and the Amplatzer occluder by US AGA have been widely used in China. And the interventional occlusion has become the main therapy of occluding the arterial duct so far.

Electronic Supplementary Material The online version of this chapter (https://doi.org/10.1007/978-981-15-2055-6_8) contains supplementary material, which is available to authorized users.

8.1 Anatomical Features

Krichenko published the first angiographic morphologic classification of PDA, classifying them into types A through E [2]. Subsequently, Phillip et al. [3] in their review of 100 children expanded the classification to name the Fetal- (F-) type PDA, comparable to Krichenko's initial description of the type C (tubular) ductus (Fig. 8.1). However, the F-type, found primarily in premature infants, differs in having a longer length and slight bend at the pulmonary arterial end. These are important characteristics when considering the possibility of transcatheter closure in this unique group of patients.

8.2 Pathophysiology

Because systemic circulation resistance is larger than pulmonary circulation resistance, aortic pressure is higher than pulmonary artery pressure in both systole and diastole, with blood continuously shunting from left to right. The shunt volume varies based on the size of pressure gradient between aorta and pulmonary artery, arterial duct diameter, and pulmonary vessel resistance. The larger the pressure gradient and PDA diameter and the smaller the pulmonary vessel resistance, the greater the shunt volume, and vice versa. In PDA, the lungs not only receive blood from the right heart but also from the left heart through the arterial duct. Therefore, blood return and volume load to left ventricle increase. The left heart compensates the shunts in lungs by increasing stroke volume which may gradually cause left ventricular hypertrophy and even failure. Because blood deviates from systemic to pulmonary circulation through the arterial duct for a long time, pulmonary circulation pressure increases, obstructing right cardiac output and gradually thickening the right ventricle. Small arteries in the lung start to manifest reflective spasm, while pulmonary hypertension worsens. This dynamic evolution continues for a long time,

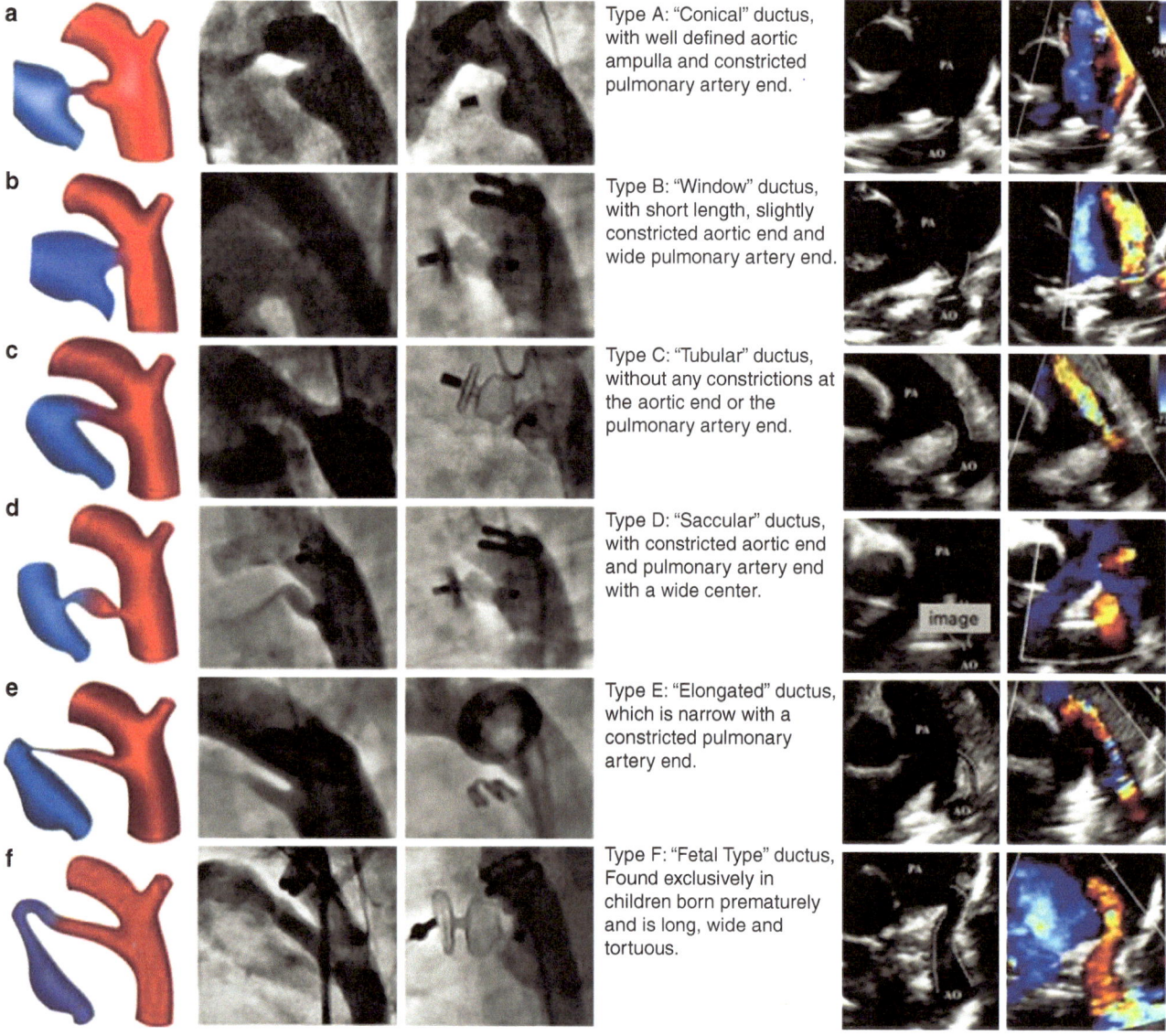

Type A: "Conical" ductus, with well defined aortic ampulla and constricted pulmonary artery end.

Type B: "Window" ductus, with short length, slightly constricted aortic end and wide pulmonary artery end.

Type C: "Tubular" ductus, without any constrictions at the aortic end or the pulmonary artery end.

Type D: "Saccular" ductus, with constricted aortic end and pulmonary artery end with a wide center.

Type E: "Elongated" ductus, which is narrow with a constricted pulmonary artery end.

Type F: "Fetal Type" ductus, Found exclusively in children born prematurely and is long, wide and tortuous.

Fig. 8.1 The modified Krichenko classification as described by Philip et al. [3] with attention to the newly named F-type ductus seen most commonly in extremely low birth weight (ELBW) infants

with pulmonary vessels experiencing secondary change which gradually develops into obstructive pulmonary arterial hypertension. Pulmonary artery pressure continuously rises and when it approaches or surpasses aortic pressure, bidirectional shunts or "right-to-left shunts" may appear. Oxyhemoglobin saturation of peripheral arterial blood decreases manifesting as cyanosis, i.e., the Eisenmenger's syndrome.

8.3   Indications and Contraindications

1. Indications
   - Left-to-right shunt, funnel and tubular type PDAs with narrowest diameter of 2–5.5 mm.
   - Age >6 months and weight >4 kg.

- No other concomitant complex congenital heart disease requiring surgery.
- Presence of residual shunt after PDA surgery.
2. Contraindications
   - Congenital heart disease that is dependent on the presence of PDA.
   - Severe pulmonary hypertension and right-to-left shunting have occurred.
   - The sepsis was not cured, and the infection was severe within 1 month before the closure.
   - Combine other cardiac malformations that require surgery.
3. PDA closure in infants
   Infants less than 1 year old, especially those younger than 6 months, have a narrower vessel and a shorter right ventricular outflow tract, increasing the difficulty of PDA

interventional therapy. Select the occluder of the size suitable for the patient, try to put the aortic side of occluder on the left side of the ampulla of the patent ductus to prevent aorta stenosis; reduce the risk of the occluder inappropriately protrudes to the left pulmonary artery to prevent left pulmonary stenosis. The procedure should be gentle and an appropriate delivery sheath is selected to avoid serious complications such as venous tears and thrombosis caused by venous tears and fractures caused by excessive sheath. If the PDA does not cause hemodynamic changes such as pulmonary hypertension, cardiac hypertrophy, cardiac dysfunction, or heart failure, the procedure can be performed at regular intervals until 1 2 years of age. In infant and child with huge PDA, surgical ligation may be safer and more effective without proper occluder selection.

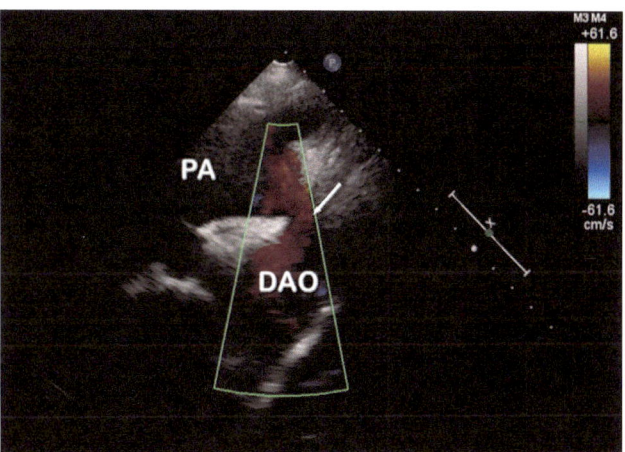

Fig. 8.2 Transthoracic echocardiography. Two-dimensional parasternal short-axis view shows patent arterial duct, allowing to measure its length and diameters of openings at aortic and pulmonary artery side. *DAO* Descending aorta, *PA* Pulmonary artery

8.4 Pre-procedural Assessment

8.4.1 Routine Assessment and Laboratory Tests

Function of heart and other organs is comprehensively evaluated using chest X-ray, electrocardiogram, echocardiography, routine blood, hepatic and renal function tests and blood electrolytes, bleeding and coagulation time, and indexes of infectious diseases. For patients with a history of respiratory system or significant thoracic deformity, pulmonary function assessment should be performed.

8.4.2 Pre-procedural TTE or TEE Assessment

The following parameters should be evaluated to assist the operator in procedural planning and device selection: the type and length of PDA, the inner diameter of PDA openings at the aortic and pulmonary artery side, and the direction of blood flow of PDA (Fig. 8.2). Previously, a minimal length of 6 mm was thought to be required to avoid the complications of left pulmonary artery stenosis and/or aortic coarctation; however, with the availability of the Piccolo device, a minimal ductal length of 3 mm may be sufficient. In our experience, the very short, "aortopulmonary window" type ducts are not well suited for percutaneous closure in this population, but fortunately the short ductus is quite rare in premature infants [4]. Poor visualization of the ductus and surrounding vasculature by echocardiography is a relative contraindication to this procedure as device placement heavily relies on adequate visualization and measurements of the ductus as well as intra-procedural assessment of the left pulmonary artery and thoracic aorta so as to minimize complications of vascular stenosis. Those with unsuitable anatomy for transcatheter closure undergo standard surgical ligation at the bedside.

8.5 Percutaneous Devices

Appropriate device selection based on PDA morphology and imaging assessment before and during deployment have proven essential to successful transcatheter PDA closure in ELBW infants. Few devices are particularly suited for PDA closure in small and preterm infants. Table 8.1 [4] provides a summary of commercially available devices in the United States that were used with some frequency in preterm and small infants for PDA closure in the recent past. While we and others were able to achieve acceptable success rates with these devices, it was apparent that a device that was smaller, came in shorter lengths, and had a softer delivery system would be advantageous for this patient population.

The ADO II device is a self-expanding device comprised of two layers of nitinol, a nickel-titanium alloy, shaped in two symmetrical retention discs and a smaller central waist frame. The maximum model is 6 mm, so it is not suitable for PDAs larger than 5.5 mm. If a ventricular septal defect occluder is used, it is not limited by the model and can block larger diameter PDAs, but it should be noted that the delivery system is also thicker and harder, and it is easy to damage the ductus artery. It has a bigger disc-to-waist ratio and is therefore not particularly well suited for PDA closure in ELBW infants as the relatively large retention discs can cause left pulmonary artery (LPA) or aortic obstruction.

The AVP II, mentioned above, is a self-expanding, multilayered, nitinol device with a symmetric frame. Outer disc

Table 8.1 Characteristics of devices commonly used for ductus arteriosus occlusion in preterm and small infants

Device				
Name	ADO II	ADO II-AS (Piccolo)	AVP II	MVP
Disc size (mm)	9–12	4–6.5	3–22	–
Waist size (mm)	3–6	3–5	3–22	5.3–13
Length (mm)	4–6	2–6	6–18	12–18
Sheath size (F)	4–5F	4F	4–7F	Microcatheter 4–5F
FDA approval	2013	2019	2007	2015

Coils are not included. *ADO* Amplatzer Duct Occluder, *ADO II-AS* Amplatzer Duct Occluder II Additional Sizes (Piccolo), *AVP* Amplatzer Vascular Plug, *MVP* Micro Vascular Plug, *FDA* Food and Drug Administration

diameter is identical to central waist diameter. It is available in small diameters (3, 4, and 6 mm) suitable for this population; however, it is only available in 6 mm lengths at these diameters. While the ELBW neonate PDA is typically long, intraductal deployment of this device relies on the exertion of external radial force to maintain stability within the PDA. This results in device lengthening, which raises the risk of LPA or aortic obstruction by the ends of the device [5]. Additionally, the delivery cable for this device is somewhat stiff, making the ultimate device position following release somewhat unpredictable in the ELBW infant.

The Medtronic micro vascular plug (MVP) is a nitinol cage-like framework covered by a polytetrafluoroethylene (PTFE) membrane which lacks retention discs, making it attractive for the tubular PDA of premature infants. It is designed for immediate vessel occlusion and predictable deployment. Its two smaller diameter devices, MVP-3Q and MVP-5Q, have a unique microcatheter delivery sheath, which is desirable for small infants. Initial results with this device in the ELBW population have been encouraging.

The ADO II-AS device (now rebranded as the Abbott Piccolo device, Abbott, MN, USA) was approved for PDA closure outside the United States for children >6 kg. This device had numerous characteristics which were desirable for PDA closure in ELBW neonates, including: availability in a variety of small diameters (3, 4, 5 mm) and short lengths (2, 4, 6 mm), retention discs only slightly larger than the central waist (Fig. 8.3) and a remarkably soft delivery cable. The Piccolo design modification is an improvement on the AVP II and the ADO II for ELBW ductal variants because the discs on the device are only slightly larger than its waist. It has a softer delivery cable than other Amplatzer self-expanding devices, which allows for much more predictable release of the device and increased application to the anatomic variants of PDA in premature infants. Following a recent multicenter trial, this device has recently been approved in the United States for closure of PDA in ELBW

infants >700 g and 3 days of age and is our device of choice for this procedure.

8.6   Procedure

Antibiotics are given intravenouously once half an hour pre-procedure. Patient should be placed in supine position. Echocardiographic examination was performed prior to procedure to reconfirm the size and length of patent duct artery. Adolescents, children, and infants should be treated under general anesthesia, and adults should be treated with 1% lidocaine local anesthesia.

After anesthesia, the right femoral artery is punctured with a 20G trocar. Distance between right femoral artery puncture site and second intercostal space of sternal left side should be measured and marked as working length. A 5F arterial sheath is inserted into the right femoral artery. A 5F pigtail catheter is adjusted to bend the distal end of catheter in 1/3 arc according to the angle between PDA and descending artery.

An echocardiographic probe was placed at suprasternal notch to reveal the aortic arch. The catheter and guide wire are advanced through the arterial sheath to the PDA. The guide wire is then pulled back and the catheter is adjusted towards the pulmonary artery. The guide wire is gently pushed into the pulmonary artery through the PDA; blind progress must be avoided. After the guide wire has passed through the PDA, the ultrasound probe is placed at the third intercostal space on the left side of the sternum to show a long-axis view of the pulmonary artery so that the guide wire in the pulmonary artery can be seen.

Leave the guide wire and remove the catheter. Catheter insertion depth was measured and a 4-5F delivery sheath (TorqVue LP delivery system, U.S.A AGA Medicine Co., Ltd.) was advanced. Under echocardiography monitoring, the catheter is advanced to the pulmonary artery through the PDA (Fig. 8.4b). The depth of insertion of the delivery sheath

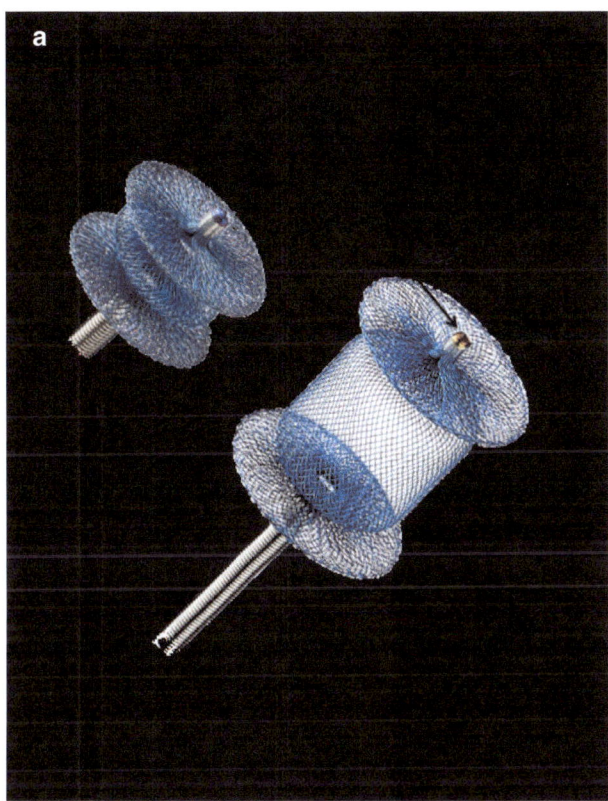

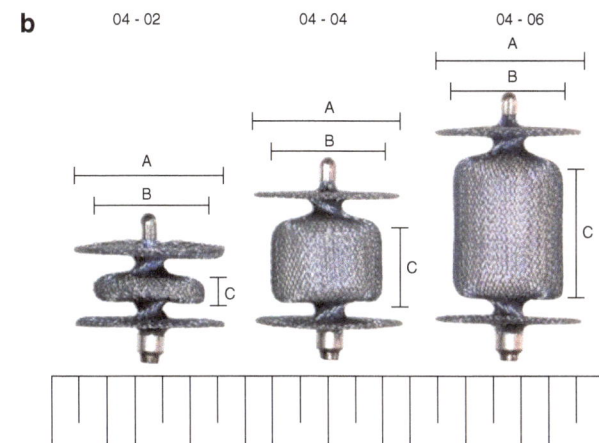

Device Name	Model/Type	A mm (in)	B mm (in)	C mm (in)
ADO II AS Occluder	9-PDA2ASIDE-03-02	4.00 (0.157)	3.00 (0.118)	2.00 (0.079)
ADO II AS Occluder	9-PDA2ASIDE-03-04	4.00 (0.157)	3.00 (0.118)	4.00 (0.157)
ADO II AS Occluder	9-PDA2ASIDE-03-06	4.00 (0.157)	3.00 (0.118)	6.00 (0.236)
ADO II AS Occluder	9-PDA2ASIDE-04-02	5.25 (0.207)	4.00 (0.157)	2.00 (0.079)
ADO II AS Occluder	9-PDA2ASIDE-04-04	5.25 (0.207)	4.00 (0.157)	4.00 (0.157)
ADO II AS Occluder	9-PDA2ASIDE-04-06	5.25 (0.207)	4.00 (0.157)	6.00 (0.236)
ADO II AS Occluder	9-PDA2ASIDE-05-02	6.50 (0.256)	5.00 (0.197)	2.00 (0.079)
ADO II AS Occluder	9-PDA2ASIDE-05-04	6.50 (0.256)	5.00 (0.197)	4.00 (0.157)
ADO II AS Occluder	9-PDA2ASIDE-05-06	6.50 (0.256)	5.00 (0.197)	6.00 (0.236)

Fig. 8.3 (**a**) High resolution photographs of the 4 mm Amplatzer Piccolo Occluder of three different lengths. (**b**) Diameters of the discs (A), and the device waist (B) and device length (C) of all nine device sizes. Note how retention discs are only slightly larger than the central waist of the device

should not exceed 3–8 cm of the depth of insertion of the pigtail catheter.

If ultrasound image is unclear, the pressure can be measured through the catheter. If the catheter enters the right ventricle too deeply, it should be pulled back slowly to the pulmonary artery under ultrasound and pressure monitoring.

The occluder should be 1–2 mm larger than the minimum PDA diameter measured by echocardiography (Fig. 8.3a).

The guide wire was withdrawn, an occluder (ADO II occluder, U.S.A. AGA Medicine Co., Ltd.) was advanced, and the aortic side of the occluder was released (Fig. 8.3c). The sheath is then pulled back to bring the occluder closer to the opening of the PDA at the pulmonary artery, releasing the remainder of the occluder under echocardiography guidance (Fig. 8.3d).

The position and shape of the occluder, residual shunt, blood flow velocity, and pulmonary artery pressure were assessed; pulmonary arterial pressure and aortic pressure were compared. After the closure is completed, turn the delivery rod counterclockwise to release the occluder. The shape and position of the occluder and blood flow velocity in the aorta and pulmonary artery should be evaluated again. If the conditions are good, remove the delivery system. The puncture site is wrapped and pressed to stop bleeding.

8.7   Method for Sealing PDA with Thrombus

In some PDA patients, echocardiographic measurements of PDA diameters >2 mm may be overestimated; after the guide wire passes through the PDA, the catheter cannot enter the pulmonary artery; strong manipulation should be avoided. Instead, the catheter should be pushed to pulmonary side of the opening of PDA and the guide wire should be properly withdrawn but still within the pulmonary artery. The guide wire and catheter should be kept in the place for 20 min. After the thrombus is formed around the guide wire, the catheter is retained and the guide wire is slowly withdrawn to seal the PDA with the thrombus. Although the immediate success rate of this strategy is as high as 80–90%, but there is the risk of re-opening of PDA.

8.8   Post-procedural Treatment

After procedure, patient should rest in bed for 24 h; ECG and vital signs, heart rate and rhythm, blood pressure and oxygen saturation should be monitored. Hematoma at puncture site and dorsalis pedis pulse should be observed periodically to avoid lower extremity ischemia by puncture site compression.

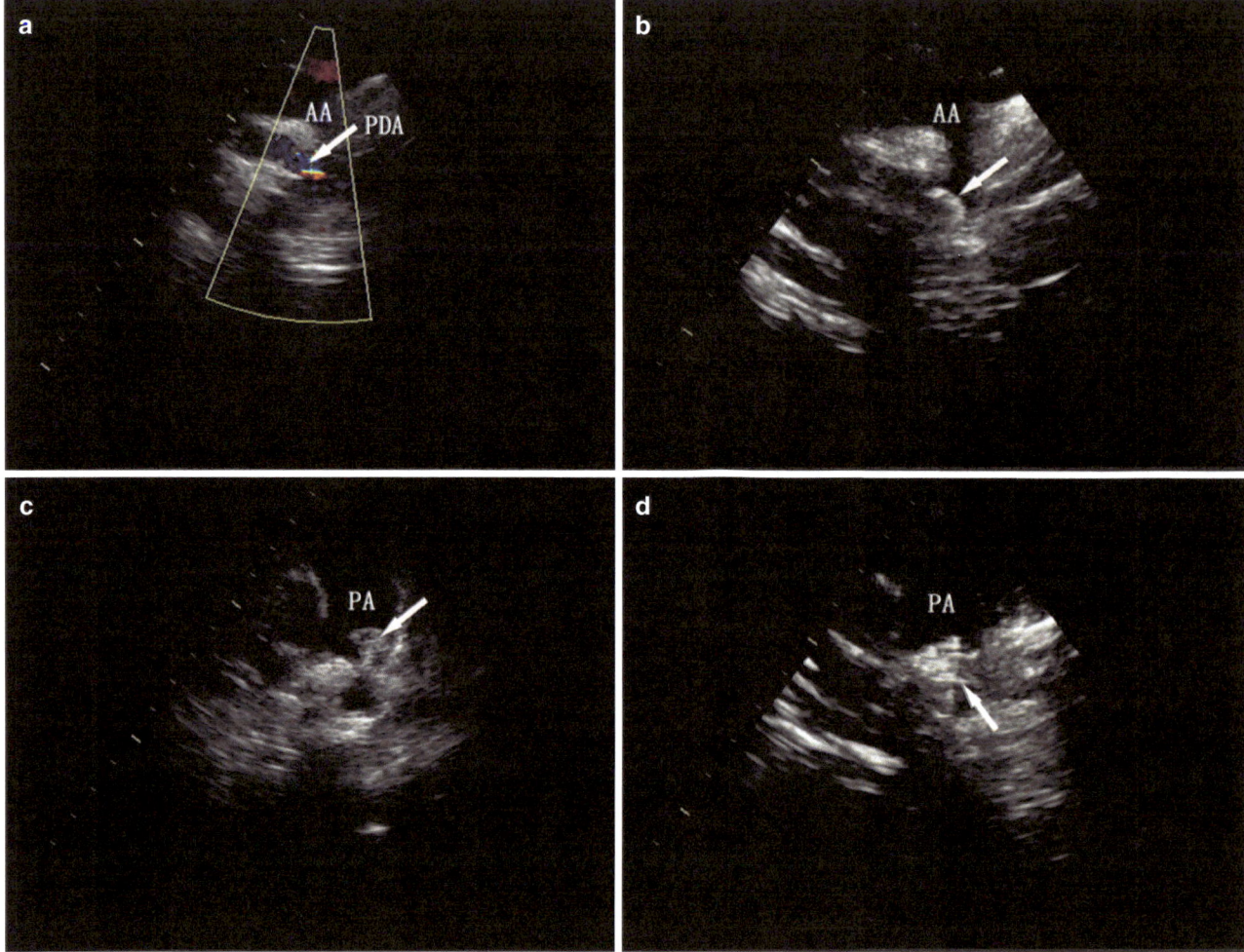

Fig. 8.4 Echocardiography-guided interventional PDA closure by femoral artery approach. (**a**) PDA (↑) diameter was measured at suprasternal view. (**b**) Suprasternal view showed the distal end of sheath (↑) through PDA. (**c**) Occluder is released in the pulmonary artery (**d**). Same view showed occluder (↑) in aortic side. *PDA* patent ductus arteriosus, *AA* Aortic arch, *PA* pulmonary artery

Intravenous antibiotic should be administered 6h post-procedure. At 24 h after procedure, echocardiography, electrocardiography, and chest X-ray should be performed. Patient should be followed up at 1, 3, 6, and 12 months and yearly after procedure with echocardiography examination to evaluate occluder location, residual shunt, including velocity of blood flow in descending aorta and left and right pulmonary arteries, and the parameters of cardiac chambers and function.

8.9   Complications and Treatment

8.9.1   Residual Shunt

Residual shunt is a major complication of PDA closure and is related to PDA type, occluder shape and displacement. Estimating residual shunt after release of the occluder during procedure is the key to correct in time. Moderate or severe residual shunts may be secondary to occluder displacement and should be treated by reclosing or surgery.

8.9.2   Occluder Displacement

An under-size occluder or improper operation usually results in displacement of the occluder, which is usually embolized into the pulmonary or abdominal aorta and its branches. The occluder can be retrieved from the pulmonary artery using a snare or foreign body tweezers; otherwise, the occluder needs to remove and ligate the PDA by surgery.

8.9.3   Hemolysis

Progressive mechanical hemolysis is a rare complication of PDA closure, but it is important. Hemolysis due to large high-speed residual shunts occurs mainly 24 h after surgery. Therefore, it is required to occlude the PDA completely during the procedure to avoid the ejection residual shunt flow. The patient's daily urine volume and color should be observed and urine routine test, hemoglobin levels, and hematocrit should be tested to observe changes. For patients with mild hemolysis, conservative treatment should be used, including alkalized urine, glucocorticoids, and appropriate blood transfusions. Most patients can recover. If conservative treatment fails or hemolysis becomes progressive, PDA ligation and removing of the occluder should be performed by surgery.

8.9.4 Stenosis of Left Pulmonary Artery and Aorta

In PDA occlusion procedure, left pulmonary stenosis is secondary to an occluder which is too long. Aortic stenosis is secondary to the use of an occluder with a larger diameter than the PDA. To avoid such complications, adjust the position or size of the occluder or select a special type of PDA occluder. After the occluder is completely released, mild stenosis may occur and regular follow-up should be performed. Stenosis is obvious, and surgical removal is required.

8.9.5 Dissection of Aorta and Pulmonary Artery

Repeated push and withdrawal of the occluder in the aorta and pulmonary artery may result in damage to the intima; if severe, it may cause aortic or pulmonary dissection. Conservative, supportive, or surgical treatment should be chosen accordingly. Avoiding repeated occlusion retraction can prevent this complication.

8.9.6 Infective Endocarditis

If there is no history of infection and fever in the first month before surgery, strict disinfection and standard operation during procedure, the infective endocarditis can generally be avoided. If fever, discomfort, myalgia, and joint pain occur after procedure, cardiac echocardiography, color Doppler examination, and blood culture are required. Appropriate antibiotic treatment should be applied as soon as possible after diagnosis.

8.10 Cases

Case 1 A 10-year-old girl, weighing 35 kg (Video 8.1).

History: The patient had a cold and fever 1 week ago. Physical examination found heart murmur, and color Doppler showed congenital heart disease—PDA. The child was prone to catch cold, but there was no history of lips cyanosis, shortness of breath, sweating, or palpitations, and there is no sig-

nificant change in body weight. She was admitted for treatment of PDA.

Physical examination: body temperature 36.3 °C, heart rate 100 beats/min, respiratory rate 24 beats/min, blood pressure 95/58 mmHg. 3/6 continuous murmurs could be heard between the second and third ribs on the left side of the sternum.

Echocardiography examination showed a patent duct artery with an inner diameter of 4 mm and a length of approximately 4 mm with a high-velocity left-to-right shunt. The electrocardiogram showed sinus rhythm, and the chest X-ray showed pulmonary congestion. The diagnosis was PDA.

Procedure: The PDA was closed by the femoral artery approach, the patient was placed in the supine position, general anesthesia, no tracheal intubation, under TTE guidance. The 5F arterial sheath was inserted after puncture of the right femoral artery. The adjusted A5F pigtail catheter and guide wire were first advanced into the descending aorta through the PDA into the pulmonary artery. The pigtail catheter was removed and the 5F delivery sheath was advanced along the guide wire into the PDA. A 6 mm × 4 mm PDA occluder (AGA) was implanted for closure. There were no residual shunts, conduction block, pericardial effusion, and hemolysis after procedure.

Case 2 A 4-year-old boy, weighing 15.5 kg (Video 8.2).

History: Physical examination found heart murmur 1 year ago, and color Doppler showed congenital heart disease—PDA. The child was prone to catch cold, but there was no history of lips cyanosis, shortness of breath, sweating, or palpitations, and there was no significant change in body weight. He was admitted for treatment of PDA.

Physical and laboratory examination: Body temperature was 36.3 °C, heart rate 115 beats/min, respiratory rate 25/min, and blood pressure 95/58 mmHg. The border of cardiac dullness was left expanded, and a 4/6 continuous murmur could be heard in the second intercostal space at left sternal border. Echocardiography examination showed that the funnel-shaped PDA has an inner diameter of 3 mm and a length of about 4 mm with a high-velocity left-to-right shunt. The electrocardiogram showed sinus arrhythmia. Chest X-ray examination was consistent with congenital heart disease, most likely PDA.

Procedure: The PDA was closed by the femoral artery approach; the patient was in the supine position with general anesthesia, no tracheal intubation, under TTE guidance. The 5F arterial sheath was inserted after puncture of the right femoral artery. The trimmed 5F pigtail catheter and guide wire were first pushed into the descending aorta through the PDA into the pulmonary artery. The pigtail catheter was removed and the 5F delivery sheath was advanced along the guide wire into the PDA. A 5 mm × 4 mm PDA occluder (AGA) was implanted for closure. There were no residual shunts, conduction block, pericardial effusion, and hemolysis after procedure.

Case 3 A 28-year-old male, weighing 74 kg (Video 8.3).

History: A heart murmur was found during physical examination half year ago, and color Doppler echocardiography showed congenital heart disease—PDA. The patient had no history of colds, cyanosis, dyspnea, malaise, sweating, or palpitations. The patient was referred to our hospital for treatment of PDA.

Physical examination and assessment: Body temperature was 36.3 °C, heart rate 68 beats/min, respiratory rate 16 times/min, and blood pressure 123/66 mmHg. A 3/6 continuous murmur was heard at the second intercostal space at left sternal border. Echocardiography revealed a funnel-shaped catheter that was 13 mm long and had a 4 mm inner diameter of the PDA opening in pulmonary artery side. There was a left-to-right shunt in pulmonary artery. The electrocardiogram showed sinus rhythm. Procedure: The PDA was closed by the femoral artery approach; the patient was in the supine position with general anesthesia, no tracheal intubation, under TTE guidance. The 5F arterial sheath was inserted after puncture of the right femoral artery. The adjusted A5F

pigtail catheter and a guide wire were first pushed into the descending aorta through the PDA into the pulmonary artery. The pigtail catheter was removed and the 5F delivery sheath was advanced along the guide wire into the PDA. A 6 mm × 4 mm PDA occluder (AGA) was implanted for closure. There were no residual shunts, conduction block, pericardial effusion, and hemolysis after procedure.

References

1. Porstmann W, Wierny L, Warnke H. [Closure of ductus arteriosus persistens without thoracotomy]. Radiol Diagn (Berl). 1968;9:168–9.
2. Krichenko A, Benson LN, Burrows P, Moes CA, McLaughlin P, Freedom RM. Angiographic classification of the isolated, persistently patent ductus arteriosus and implications for percutaneous catheter occlusion. Am J Cardiol. 1989;63:877–80.
3. Philip R, Waller BR 3rd, Agrawal V, et al. Morphologic characterization of the patent ductus arteriosus in the premature infant and the choice of transcatheter occlusion device. Catheter Cardiovasc Interv. 2016;87:310–7.
4. Almeida-Jones M, Tang NY, Reddy A, Zahn E. Overview of transcatheter patent ductus arteriosus closure in preterm infants. Congenit Heart Dis. 2019;14:60–4.
5. Zahn EM, Peck D, Phillips A, et al. Transcatheter closure of patent ductus arteriosus in extremely premature newborns: early results and midterm follow-up. JACC Cardiovasc Interv. 2016;9:2429–37.

9.1 Anatomical Features

Krichenko published the first angiographic morphologic classification of PDA, classifying them into types A through E. Subsequently, Phillip et al. in their review of 100 children expanded the classification to name the Fetal- (F-) type PDA, comparable to Krichenko's initial description of the type C (tubular) ductus. However, the F-type, found primarily in premature infants, differs in having a longer length and slight bend at the pulmonary arterial end. These are important characteristics when considering the possibility of transcatheter closure in this unique group of patients.

9.2 Pathophysiology

Because systemic circulation resistance is larger than pulmonary circulation resistance, aortic pressure is higher than pulmonary artery pressure in both systole and diastole, with blood continuously shunting from left to right. The shunt volume varies based on the size of pressure gradient between aorta and pulmonary artery, arterial duct diameter, and pulmonary vessel resistance. The larger the pressure gradient and PDA diameter and the smaller the pulmonary vessel resistance, the greater the shunt volume, and vice versa. In PDA, the lungs not only receive blood from the right heart but also from the left heart through the arterial duct. Therefore, blood return and volume load to left ventricle increase. The left heart compensates the shunts in lungs by increasing stroke volume which may gradually cause left ventricular hypertrophy and even failure. Because blood deviates from systemic to pulmonary circulation through the arterial duct for a long time, pulmonary circulation pressure increases, obstructing right cardiac output and gradually

thickening the right ventricle. Small arteries in the lung start to manifest reflective spasm, while pulmonary hypertension worsens. This dynamic evolution continues for a long time, with pulmonary vessels experiencing secondary change which gradually develops into obstructive pulmonary arterial hypertension. Pulmonary artery pressure continuously rises and when it approaches or surpasses aortic pressure, bidirectional shunts or "right-to-left shunts" may appear. Oxyhemoglobin saturation of peripheral arterial blood decreases manifesting as cyanosis, i.e., the Eisenmenger's syndrome.

9.3 Indications and Contraindications

9.3.1 Indications

- Funnel and tubular PDA with a minimum internal diameter of 2–14 mm, with left-to-right shunt. The patients with PDA inner diameter ≥4 mm are more suitable for interventional closure through femoral vein approach [1].
- Weight >7 kg.
- There are no other complex congenital heart diseases that require surgery.
- Patients with residual shunt after PDA closure procedure.

9.3.2 Contraindications

- Congenital heart disease that is dependent on PDA.
- Severe pulmonary artery hypertension with right-to-left shunt.
- Sepsis was not completely treated and a serious infection occurred within 1 month before closure.
- PDA diameter >14 mm (if the diameter of PDA is too large, the procedure is technically challenging, the success rate is low and the complication rate is high) [2].

Electronic Supplementary Material The online version of this chapter (https://doi.org/10.1007/978-981-15-2055-6_9) contains supplementary material, which is available to authorized users.

9.3.3   Huge PDA

Interventional therapy in patients with giant PDA is techni-cally challenging, especially infants, and can lead to descend-ing aortic stenosis and hemolysis, as well as other complications. The key is to choose the right sealing equip-ment. Consider the PDA diameter, shape, and risks of shed-ding, rupture, and more. The most commonly used PDA occluder is typically used for PDA diameters ≤11 mm. For PDA with a diameter >11 mm, Huang et al. reported the use of atrial septal defect (ASD) occluder to close PDA, but the residual shunt rate was higher. Thanopoulos et al. reported that the Amplatzer ventricular septal defect (VSD) occluder was used to close large PDA in patients with severe pulmo-nary hypertension and got good results. For the patients with large internal diameter of PDA especially those with severe pulmonary hypertension, who are prone to suffering pulmo-nary dissection during procedure, repeated deploying and retracting of the occluder should be avoided. Surgical liga-tion should be selected for high-risk patients.

9.4   Pre-procedural Preparation

9.4.1   Routine Assessment and Laboratory Tests

Function of heart and other organs is comprehensively evalu-ated using chest X-ray, electrocardiogram, echocardiogra-phy, routine blood, hepatic and renal function tests and blood electrolytes, bleeding and coagulation time, and indexes of infectious diseases. For patients with a history of respiratory system or significant thoracic deformity, pulmonary function assessment should be performed.

9.4.2   Pre-procedural TTE or TEE Assessment

The following parameters should be evaluated to assist the operator in procedural planning and device selection: the type and length of PDA, the inner diameter of PDA openings at the aortic and pulmonary artery side, and the direction of blood flow of PDA. Previously, a minimal length of 6 mm

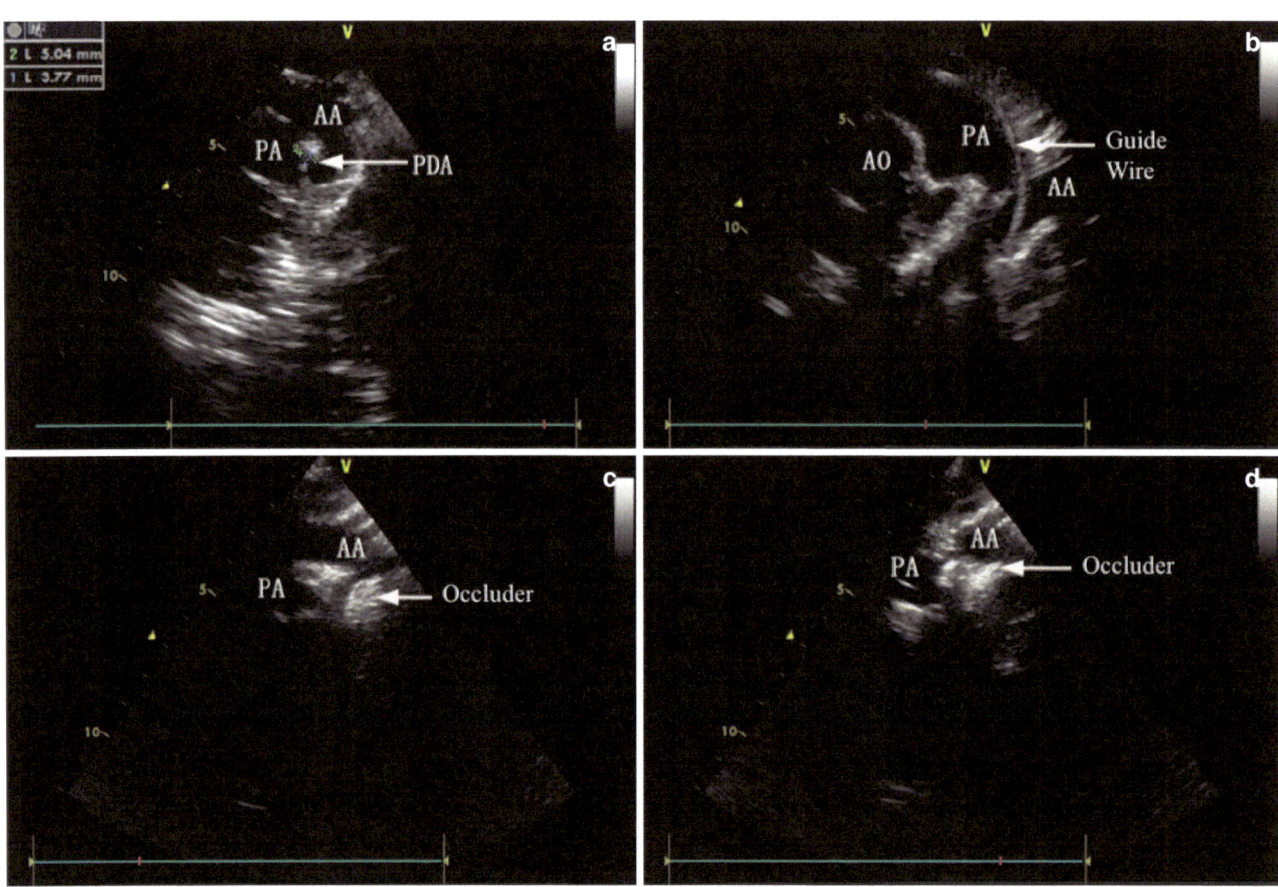

Fig. 9.1 Transthoracic echocardiography of interventional PDA clo-sure by femoral vein approach: (**a**) The suprasternal view shows the PDA (↑) diameter. (**b**) Parasternal long-axis view shows the guide wire (↑) in pulmonary artery through PDA. (**c**) The occluder (↑) was deployed at aortic side. (**d**) The occluder (↑) was deployed at the pulmo-nary artery side. *PDA* Patent ductus arteriosus, *AA* Aortic arch, *PA* Pulmonary artery, *AO* Aorta

was thought to be required to avoid the complications of left pulmonary artery stenosis and/or aortic coarctation; however, with the availability of the Piccolo device, a minimal ductal length of 3 mm may be sufficient. In our experience, the very short, "aortopulmonary window" type ducts are not well suited for percutaneous closure in this population, but fortunately the short ductus is quite rare in premature infants. Poor visualization of the ductus and surrounding vasculature by echocardiography is a relative contraindication to this procedure as device placement heavily relies on adequate visualization and measurements of the ductus as well as intra-procedural assessment of the left pulmonary artery and thoracic aorta so as to minimize complications of vascular stenosis. Those with unsuitable anatomy for transcatheter closure undergo standard surgical ligation at the bedside.

9.5 Procedure

- Echocardiography should be performed to reconfirm the diameter and length of the PDA before procedure (Fig. 9.1a). The patient should be in the supine position. Adolescents, children, and infants should be under general anesthesia with spontaneous breathing. One percent lidocaine can be used for local anesthesia in adults.
- Under anesthesia, the distance between the third intercostal space on right border of sternal and the puncture site of right femoral vein is measured and marked on the catheter as working length. A 6F sheath is inserted through the femoral vein, and a 6F right coronary catheter or pigtail catheter is delivered through the sheath. Once the catheter enters into the body and has covered the working length, it can be rotated to facilitate the echocardiography to explore its position in the right atrium and prevent it being inserted too deep and damaging the superior vena cava during rotation.
- Under echocardiography-guidance, the catheter and guide wire are advanced into right ventricle through tricuspid valve. Echocardiography allows only one portion to be inspected at a time, making it difficult to clearly determine the position of the catheter and guide wire. However, the pigtail catheter can be advanced to the working length in the right atrium, and the proximal end of the catheter is bulky and the position of the catheter is easily detected. So, we can firstly make the pigtail catheter cover the working length, and enter the right atrium, then use the curvature of the pigtail catheter to gently push the guide wire into the right ventricle. Be careful to avoid damage to the tricuspid valve and the chordae.
- The catheter is adjusted so that the top of catheter turns towards the right ventricular outflow tract, the guide wire is gently sent into the pulmonary artery through the pul-

monary valve, and the catheter is sent into the pulmonary artery along the guide wire. Then, the guide wire is withdrawn, and the pulmonary artery pressure is measured.
- The right coronary catheter is withdrawn and a multipurpose catheter (MPA2) is delivered along the guide wire, the depth of which is consistent with the insertion depth of the right coronary catheter. The main pulmonary artery and arterial catheter are displayed on the long-axis view of the main pulmonary artery in the transthoracic echocardiography. The direction of the multipurpose catheter (MPA2) is rotated and adjusted to allow the guide wire to enter the descending aorta through the PDA (Fig. 9.1b). Echocardiography should show the descending aorta through the super sternal fossa view and determine the guide wire is in the descending aorta.
- According to the diameter of the PDA measured by preoperative echocardiography, add 4–6 mm to select the occluder and the corresponding delivery system. Connect it to the front end of the delivery rod, pull back the delivery rod, put the occluder into the loading sheath, and flush with normal saline to remove the gas in the occluder and its loading sheath. Rinse the long sheath with heparin saline to ensure that the sheath is unobstructed and free of gases and blood clots.
- The multifunctional catheter (MPA2) and the sheath are withdrawn and the delivery sheath are advanced along the guide wire. The depth of the delivery sheath is 5–8 cm longer than that of the multifunctional catheter (MPA2). Then, the delivery sheath inner core and the guide wire are withdrawn.
- The occlusion device is fed along the delivery sheath. The occluder is advanced from the delivery sheath to the descending aorta to open the aortic side disc of occluder, and the occluder is slowly retracted to the aortic side of the PDA, embedded in the aortic end of the catheter, and the delivery sheath is retracted. The waist of the device is placed in the middle of PDA and observed for obvious waist sign (Fig. 9.1c, d).
- Residual shunts and velocities in the aortic arch and left and right pulmonary arteries are assessed by TTE. After confirming that the PDA is properly closed, rotate the delivery catheter counter clockwise, release the occluder, and withdraw the delivery system. Bandage the site of puncture and press bandage to stop bleeding [3–5].

9.6 Post-procedural Care

Post-procedure, the patients should rest in bed for 12 h; local compression of sandbags on the puncture site for 4 h. Blood pressure, heart rate and rhythm, and oxygen saturation should be monitored for 24 h. Antibiotics are given intravenously once half an hour pre-procedure and 6 h post-procedure, ECG and echocardiography examination should be performed within 24 h after procedure. The patients should be followed up at 1, 3, 6 months to 1 year with echocardiography examination, if necessary, take X-ray films.

9.7 Complications

9.7.1 Occluder Displacement

The incidence of occluder displacement was approximately 0.3%, mainly due to improper selection of occluder size and improper procedure. When advancing the delivery sheath, the sheath should not be rotated to avoid displacement of the occluder. Once the occluder is dropped, it should be removed using a mesh basket or foreign body forceps; otherwise, emergency surgery should be performed.

9.7.2 Hemolysis

The incidence of hemolysis is <0.8%, mainly due to excessive residual flow, or the occluder protrudes into the aorta side, and should be avoided as much as possible. Once hemolysis occurs, hemostatic agents, glucocorticoids, sodium bicarbonate, and other drugs can be used to protect kidney function. Most patients may heal by themselves. One or more occluders (usually coils) can be used for patients with a large amount of residual shunts. If hemolysis cannot be controlled by medicine therapy or the patient has persistent fever, hemolytic anemia or severe jaundice, surgery is required.

9.7.3 Residual Shunt and Occluder Displacement

Incidence of residual shunt by using mushroom occluders is ≤0.1%. One or more coils can be used to block residual shunts. Surgery should be performed if necessary. Incidence of occluder displacement is 0.4%. If residual shunt is obvious or normal cardiac structure is affected after displacement, the occluder should be surgically removed.

9.7.4 Descending Aorta Stenosis

With a mushroom occluder, the incidence of descending aortic stenosis is approximately 0.2%. It occurs primarily in infants because many occluders protrude excessively into the descending aorta, which can be avoided by careful echocardiography monitoring during the procedure. Mild stenosis (a narrow pressure difference <20 mmHg) can be closely observed. For severe stenosis, surgery should be considered.

9.7.5 Left Pulmonary Artery Stenosis

In patients using mushroom occluders, the incidence of left pulmonary stenosis was 0.2%, mainly due to the occluder extending into the pulmonary artery. This complication can be avoided by selecting a properly PDA occluder. Mild stenosis can be closely observed, and severe stenosis should be treated by surgery.

9.7.6 Tricuspid Valve Injury

When preforming the echocardiography-guided transfemoral vein intervention for the treatment of PDA, the delivery system needs to be delivered from the femoral vein through the right atrium-tricuspid-right ventricle-pulmonary artery approach access, the tricuspid valves and chordae might be damaged in the process. If resistance is encountered during the passage of the catheter, the catheter may be blocked by the tricuspid chordae. At this time, the guide wire should be fed, and the pigtail catheter should be straightened before attempting to adjust the direction of the catheter. During the procedure, the principle of gently operating should be followed to avoid damage to the tricuspid valve.

9.7.7 Pain in the Precordial Area

In patients with mushroom occluders, the incidence of chest tightness and pain was 0.3%. This is caused by the implanted occluder, which is so large that the occlude expanded and stretched the PDA and surrounding tissue. In general, this symptom may disappear over time.

9.7.8 Infective Endocarditis

Most patients with PDA have low immune function and are prone to recurrent respiratory infections. If the sterilization is not strict, the operation time is too long, and the perioperative antibiotics are improperly applied, it may cause infective endocarditis. Sterile disinfection of the catheter room, standard operation, and postoperative antibiotics are powerful measures to prevent infective endocarditis.

9.8 Summary

The use of femoral vein access in PDA closure not only reduces the risk of femoral artery injury, but also reduces the cost and duration of operation, with good safety and effectiveness. However, this technique is challenging and requires a long learning curve. In conventional interventional techniques, the position of the catheter can be easily displayed by X-rays. While echocardiography can only display a single view, and sometimes it does not accurately display the position of the catheter. In addition, the catheter and guide wire need to be rotated through large angles for two times to pass through the tricuspid valve and the pulmonary valve. The technique of interventional closure of the PDA through the femoral vein approach is more difficult than the echocardiography-guided femoral artery approach. Our experience is that the closure of the femoral vein is more suitable for patients with PDA diameter ≥4 mm. Femoral artery closure is more suitable for patients with funnel-shaped PDA with a diameter ≤4 mm in the pulmonary artery side. Interventional closure of the PDA under the guidance of echocardiography can avoid radioactive exposure. Although the technology has high requirements for operators, the highly trained team is fully qualified. This technique combined with echocardiography-guided transfemoral artery PDA closure has made the echocardiography-guided percutaneous PDA closure a promising development and application prospect.

9.9 Case

A 3-year-old girl, weighing 15 kg (Video 9.1).

Chief complaint: Found a heart murmur for 1 year.

Current medical history: The patient went to the local children's hospital for a "cold, fever" 1 year ago, and found a heart murmur.

The child is susceptible to cold, no history of lip cyanosis, dyspnea, fatigue, sweating, palpitations, and other discomfort. Physical examination: body temperature 36.3 °C, pulse 90 beats/min, breathing 24 beats/min, blood pressure 110/60 mmHg, the border of cardiac dullness was slightly left extended, and a 3/6 continuous machinery murmur could be heard at the second intercostal space along the left sternal border.

Echocardiography: The diameter of the aortic side of the arterial duct was 10 mm, the diameter of the pulmonary artery was 6 mm, and the total length was about 6 mm. It was funnel-shaped with a high-speed left-to-right shunt. The electrocardiogram showed sinus rhythm, and the chest X-ray showed pulmonary congestion, which was considered to be PDA.

Procedure: Treatment of the PDA with TTE guided by the femoral vein method. The patient was in the supine position and general anesthesia without trachea cannula. Under the guidance of TTE, the 6F sheath was inserted after the right femoral vein punctured. A 6F multifunctional catheter (MPA2) with a guide wire was advanced through the tricuspid valve into the pulmonary artery and into the descending aorta through the PDA. The catheter was then withdrawn and the 8F delivery sheath was advanced along the guide wire through the PDA into the descending aorta. The 12 mm PDA occluder was used for closure, and there was no postoperative complication.

References

1. El-Said HG, et al. Safety of percutaneous patent ductus arteriosus closure: an unselected multicenter population experience. J Am Heart Assoc. 2013;2(6):e000424.
2. Magee AG, et al. Transcatheter coil occlusion of the arterial duct; results of the European registry. Eur Heart J. 2001;22(19):1817–21.
3. Sungur M, et al. Closure of patent ductus arteriosus in children, small infants, and premature babies with Amplatzer duct occluder II additional sizes: multicenter study. Catheter Cardiovasc Interv. 2013;82(2):245–52.
4. Wang SZ, Liu Y, Shan W, et al. Application research of percutaneous patent ductus arteriosus closure by femoral vein approach under echocardiography guidance. Nat Med J China. 2015;95(27):2183–5.
5. Rao PS, et al. Follow-up results of transvenous occlusion of patent ductus arteriosus with the buttoned device. J Am Coll Cardiol. 1999;33(3):820–6.

Echocardiography-Guided Percutaneous Interventions for Pulmonary Valve Stenosis

10.1 Anatomical Features

Pulmonary stenosis (PS) accounts for about 8–10% of congenital heart disease. The normal pulmonary valve consists of three semi-monthly cups with free edge and its annulus attached to the myocardium of right ventricular funnel.

10.1.1 Typical Pulmonary Stenosis

The pulmonary valve is structurally intact, the leaflets become short, thick and stiff resulting in an open petal in the shape of a fish-mouth. Typically, the opening is located in the center of the annulus, or sometimes on one side. It may also be a congenital uni-or bicuspid pulmonary valve with a dome-shaped opening. The pulmonary valve annulus develops normally. The pulmonary trunk is post-stenotic dilated, and the degree of dilation is not proportional to the severity of the stenosis.

10.1.2 Dysplasia Pulmonary Stenosis

This type accounts for about 10% of pulmonary stenosis. Pulmonary valve leaflet with irregular shape is thickening or nodular but no adhesion between the leaflets. There is leaflets dysplasia, mild or none dilated pulmonary artery. Patients with this type often have a family history.

The secondary changes of the disease are right ventricular hypertrophy, myocardial ischemia, thickened tricuspid valve, Additionally, a few patients present left ventricular hypertrophy, enlarged right atrial secondary to stenosis, and patent foramen oval or ASD [1].

Electronic Supplementary Material The online version of this chapter (https://doi.org/10.1007/978-981-15-2055-6_10) contains supplementary material, which is available to authorized users.

10.2 Pathophysiology

Pulmonary stenosis leads to an increase in right ventricular pressure. In patients with severe PS, cardiac output is reduced and peripheral cyanosis and syncope may occur. In patients with pulmonary stenosis and associated with ASD or PFO, an increased right atrial pressure results in a right-to-left atrial shunt, and patients may have central cyanosis and hypoxia. Long-term and excessive right ventricular changes including increased afterload, concentric hypertrophy, subendocardial ischemia, and myocardial strain may lead to right ventricular failure.

High velocity of the blood flow through the stenotic pulmonary valve results in post-stenotic dilatation of the pulmonary artery. Pulmonary stenosis is diagnosed if the pressure gradient is greater than 20 mmHg. The degree of the pressure gradient between the right ventricle and the pulmonary artery depends on the severity of pulmonary stenosis, which can be divided into mild, moderate, and severe (Table 10.1).

10.3 Indications and Contraindications

10.3.1 Definite Indications

- Typical pulmonary valve stenosis. Patients with a normal cardiac output but pressure gradient ≥ 50 mmHg.
- Patients with dyspnea on exertion, syncope, pre-syncope, and other symptoms. The pressure gradient is ≥ 30 mmHg.

Table 10.1 Severity of pulmonary stenosis

	Mild	Moderate	Severe
Pressure gradient between right ventricle and pulmonary artery (mmHg)	<50	50–79	≥80

© Peking University Medical Press 2020
X. Pan et al., *Percutaneous and Non-fluoroscopical (PAN) Procedure for Structural Heart Disease*,
https://doi.org/10.1007/978-981-15-2055-6_10

10.3.2   Relative Indications

- Severe PS with right-to-left atrial shunt.
- Mild and moderate dysplasia PS.
- Palliative treatment (transthoracic balloon pulmonary val-vuloplasty) is recommended for infants and young children who have other complex congenital heart disease to reduce cyanosis. The fully corrected operation cannot be performed due to poor physical condition.
- Pulmonary atresia with intact ventricular septum, normal right atrial development, or mild dysplasia.
- Severe PS with small and insufficient left ventricular. Balloon valvuloplasty can be performed step by step in several times.

10.3.3   Contraindications

- Infundibular PS.
- Subvalvular PS.
- Supravalvular PS.
- Severe dysplasia PS.
- Infants with severe PS who have severe right ventricular dysplasia or right heart failure.
- Extremely severe PS or complete pulmonary atresia with intact ventricular septum with right ventricular-dependent coronary circulation.
- Age and weight are not absolute contraindications for infants in critical condition.

10.4   Pre-procedural Preparation

- Diagnosis should be determined by medical history and auxiliary examination. Before surgery, echocardiography, chest X-ray, electrocardiogram, blood test, and other auxiliary tests should be performed. Echocardiography is the most important tool for assessing structural abnormalities. The condition of the pulmonary valve can be clearly observed in parasternal long, short-axis and subcostal views. The pulmonary valve annulus should be measured to determine whether there is annulus dysplasia and choose balloon catheter. The pressure gradient of pulmonary valve can be calculated using the modified Bernoulli formula: $\Delta P = 4\, V2$. ΔP is the pressure gradient, and V is the peak velocity measured by Doppler in the pulmonary artery.
- Prostaglandin $E1$ [0.1–0.4 μg/(kg min)] is recommended for patients with extremely severe stenosis, obvious cyanosis, or severe hypoxemia with metabolic acidosis to relief symptom.
- The patients with heart failure should be effectively treated to improve cardiac function.
- Selection of interventional device

Balloon size: The ratio of balloon/annulus is recommended 1.2–1.4. Small ratio is selected for patient with severe stenosis. Relatively large ratio (1.4–1.5 times) for valve dysplasia can achieve good results.

Balloon length: 20 mm for newborns and babies; 30 mm for children; and 40 mm for adolescents and adults.

- Informed consent: Long-term prognosis is little known, and there is a risk of restenosis at long-term follow-up. Therefore, the patient and his or her family or guardians should be informed of the risks and complications that may occur. The informed consent must be signed.

10.5   Procedure

- Transpulmonary pressure gradient should be measured by pre-procedural TTE.
- Patients should be in supine position.

  For patients with high-quality TTE images, local anesthesia and sedatives should be used; general anesthesia is used for infants who are unable to cooperate. For patients who do not have high-quality TTE images and require TEE guidance, general anesthesia and endotracheal intubation should be given. Figures 10.1 and 10.2 showed images of TTE and TEE guidance, respectively.
- Marking working length. Before procedure, the distance between the right parasternal third intercostal space and the right femoral vein puncture site should be measured and marked on the catheter. When the catheter enters the body and reaches the working length, the catheter can be rotated to facilitate the echocardiography to detect the position of the catheter in the right atrium.
- The right femoral vein is punctured and a sheath is inserted (6 Fr sheath is used when the weight of the patient was less than 12 kg. The patient's body weight is more than 12 kg and 7 Fr sheath was used). Heparin (80–100 U/kg) is administered after inserting sheath.
- The guide wire and the 6F multipurpose catheter (MPA2) are delivered through the sheath, and the proximal end of guide wire is extended 2–4 cm from the catheter. The catheter and guide wire are gently pushed until the working length. The position of the catheter and the tip of the guide wire were not easily identifiable by the 2D Echo. Therefore, we suggested that the catheter can be advanced to the right atrium with the length not exceeding the working length. After reaching the working length, the guide wire is removed. Then, the catheter is gently rotated clockwise towards the right ventricular inflow tract, and it is advanced through the tricuspid valve into the right ventricle under four-chamber view. After measuring the right ventricular pressure, the catheter is rotated towards the pulmonary artery to facilitate advancement of the guide wire into the pulmonary artery via the pulmonary valve under aortic short-axis view guidance.

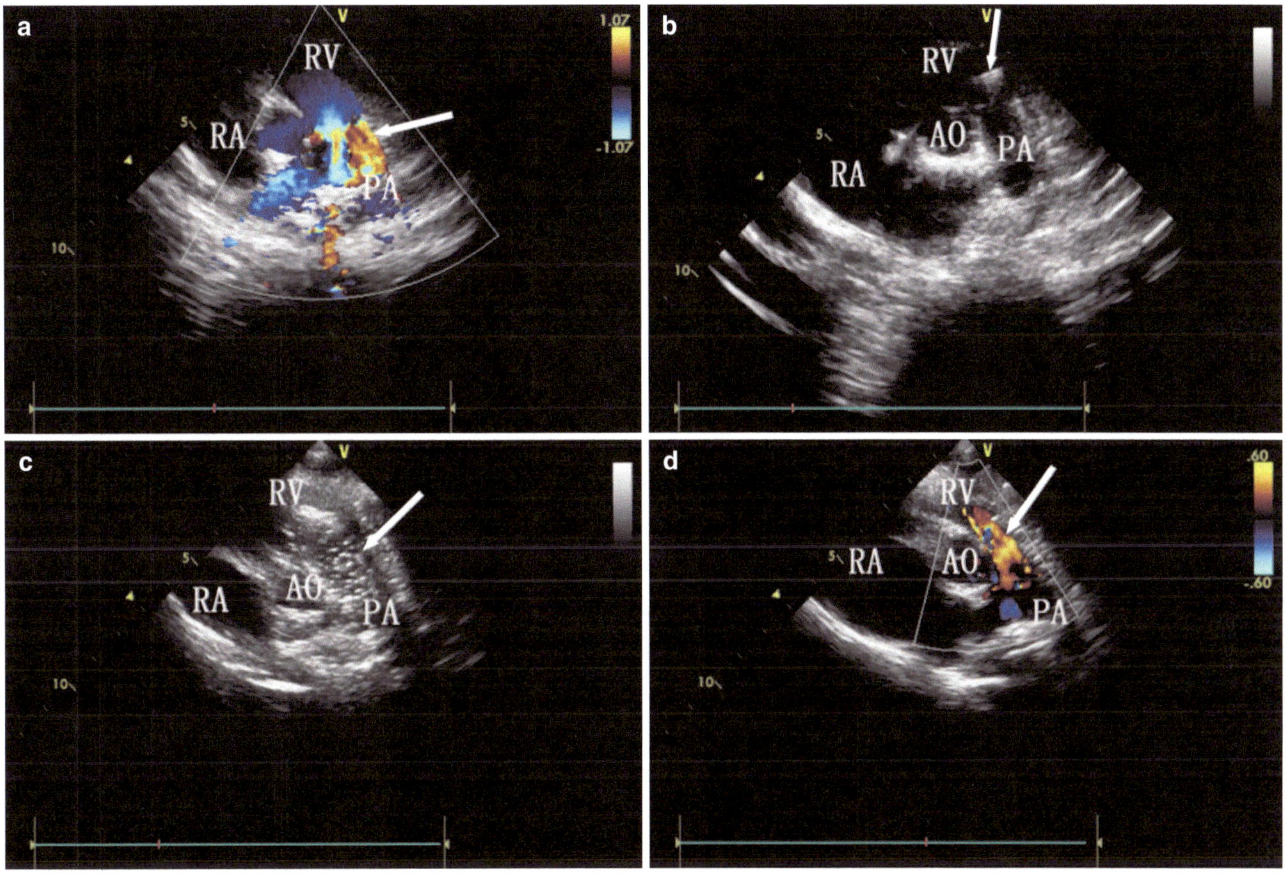

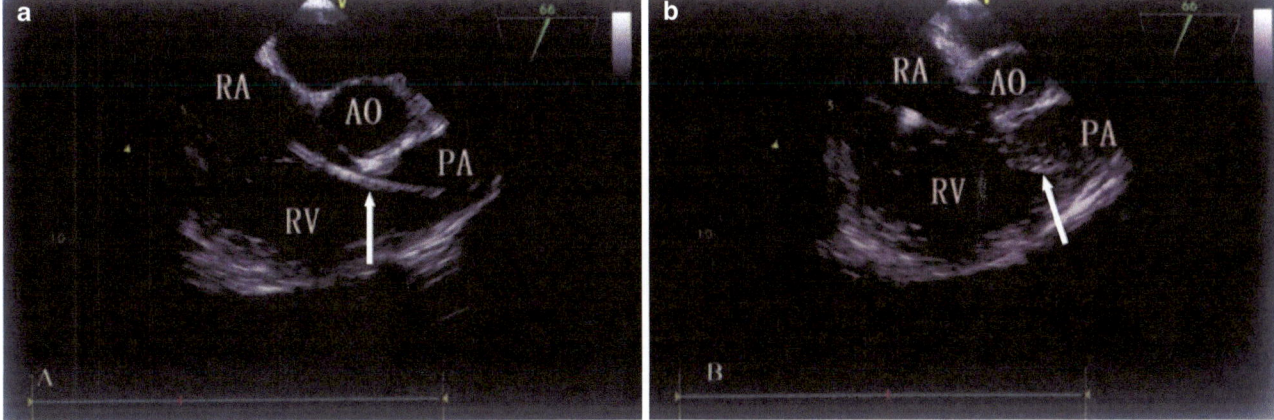

Fig. 10.1 Transthoracic echocardiography: (**a**) Parasternal short-axis view with color Doppler shows a high-velocity flow (↑) in pulmonary artery. (**b**) Same view shows the guide wire (↑) in pulmonary artery. (**c**) Same view showed the balloon (↑) is inflated with microbubble saline. (**d**) Same view with color Doppler showed a normal velocity of blood flow (↑) through pulmonary valve after valvuloplasty. *PA* Pulmonary artery, *RA* Right atrium, *RV* Right ventricle, *AO* Aorta

Fig. 10.2 Transesophageal echocardiography: (**a**) The distal end of guide wire is in pulmonary artery from right atrium through tricuspid valve, right ventricle, and pulmonary valve. (**b**) The balloon (↑) is inflated. *PA* Pulmonary artery, *RA* Right atrium, *RV* Right ventricle, *AO* Aorta

The experienced operator can use right coronary artery catheter. Swan-Ganz catheter is recommended when it is difficult for the right coronary catheter passing through pulmonary artery. However, passing the Swan-Ganz catheter through the narrow pulmonary valve may be difficult and increase costs.

- After measuring right ventricle and pulmonary artery pressure, the length of catheter inserted into the body should be measured. The super-stiff guide wire is inserted into catheter, and the catheter is withdrawn. The balloon with 1.2–1.5 times of the diameter of the pulmonary valve annulus is advanced along the guide wire. After the balloon catheter is inserted to the distance the guiding catheter was once inserted, the proximal end of the balloon can be detected in the right ventricular outflow tract by echocardiography. The balloon is advanced into pulmonary valve annulus and can be partially inflated with microbubble saline with the pressure no more than one atmospheric pressure. The position of the balloon can clearly be showed by echocardiography to adjust the balloon in the center of pulmonary valve annulus. The distal end of the balloon must be kept away from the tricuspid valve to avoid damage.

- When the balloon and the guide wire are fixed, the balloon is rapidly inflated with normal saline. As the balloon cavity increases (5–8 atmospheres), the waist sign disappears. Once the waist sign disappears, the normal saline is immediately withdrawn. The balloon is inflated for 5–10 s and reflated for 2–4 times. Sometimes, one effective inflation can achieve therapeutic purposes. In order to prevent the balloon rupture, the filling pressure of the balloon should be lower than the burst pressure specified by the manufacturer, and it should be checked carefully. The pressure should be maintained continuously until the waist sign of the balloon disappeared. To shorten the hypotension time, the inflation time should be as short as possible, usually ending when the waist sign has just disappeared. One more inflation is needed after the waist sign disappeared to ensure the valvuloplasty effect.
- After withdrawing the balloon, an multipurpose catheter (MPA2) is advanced along the guide wire to measure the pressure of pulmonary artery and right ventricle. If the pressure gradient is still greater than 40 mmHg, a second dilatation was performed with a larger balloon. If the transvalvular pressure gradient is ≤25 mmHg, which indicate that the valvuloplasty is effective. In some symptom-relieved patients (mostly severe pulmonary stenosis) who has no obvious stenosis in the right ventricle funnel with the oxygen saturation is ≤80%, modified B-T shunt should be performed.
- If the pressure gradient is satisfactory, the guide wire and catheter are withdrawn and the pulmonary regurgitation is evaluated by echocardiography.
- Withdraw the sheath, bandage the site of puncture and press bandage to stop bleeding [2–4].

10.6   Post-procedural Treatment

- A sandbag is used to compress femoral vein puncture site for 4 h, and patient should rest in bed for 12 h.
- Intravenous antibiotic is administered prophylactically for 2 days.

- All patients are followed up with echocardiography, chest radiography, and electrocardiography at 24 h, 1, 3, and 6 months, and yearly thereafter.

10.7   Complications and Treatment [5]

10.7.1 General Procedural Complications

Such as anesthesia accidents, infections, and vascular injury.

10.7.2 Pulmonary Valve Annulus Tearing and Cardiac Rupture

Mostly due to the over-sized balloon or overestimation of the annulus diameter. Once the pericardial effusion is detected by echocardiography during the procedure, the surgery should be performed immediately. If the pulmonary artery annulus is ruptured, it should be repaired by surgery under cardiopulmonary bypass.

10.7.3 Right Ventricular Tear, Hemorrhage

The majority of them occurred in neonates or low-body weight infants with weak myocardial tissue and surgical repair should be performed immediately if happened.

10.7.4 Right Ventricular Outflow Tract Spasm

Most of them are reactive spasm caused by repeated violent operation at the right ventricular outflow tract, which can lead to death in severe cases. Therefore, the procedure should be gently performed, if the spasm occurs, the procedure should be suspended and resumed after spasm is relieved. A β-blockers, such as propranolol, can be used if necessary.

10.7.5 Transient Response

During the inflation, the right ventricular outflow tract is blocked by the balloon, causing blood pressure reduction, bradycardia, hypoxia, etc. Once the balloon is deflated, these symptoms disappear.

10.7.6 Apnea

Due to balloon inflation time is too long or too frequent.

10.7.7 Arrhythmia

During the valvuloplasty procedure, the transient complete atrioventricular block or tachyarrhythmia may occur, which will disappear after withdraw device.

10.7.8 Post-procedural Pulmonary Valve Restenosis

The valvuloplasty can be performed again to alleviate recurrence or residual stenosis, but it is necessary to determine the cause of restenosis before surgery. Surgical therapy is recommended for patients with severe PS and an associated hypoplastic pulmonary annulus, severe pulmonary regurgitation, subvalvular PS, or supravalvular PS [6].

In order to prevent the above complications, the following should be noted:

1. Strictly control the indications.
2. The anatomy and pathophysiology of pulmonary stenosis need to be comprehensively evaluated before surgery.
3. The balloon should be selected according to the guideline.
4. The hemodynamics, blood oxygen saturation, acid-base, and electrolyte balance should be closely monitored during and after surgery.
5. The vital signs should be closely monitored after the procedure and the echocardiography should be performed within 2 h after procedure, if necessary.

10.8 Cases

Case 1 Patient was 3.6 years old, male, weighing 14.5 kg (Video 10.1), found a heart murmur for more than 1 year. No history of lip cyanosis, syncope, swelling, or hemoptysis. His development was normal. Echocardiography suggested: moderate pulmonary valve stenosis, the transvalvular pressure gradient was 58 mmHg, and the diameter of pulmonary valve annulus was 13 mm. The pulmonary valvuloplasty through the femoral vein was performed under the guidance of echocardiography.

The right femoral vein was punctured; a 9F sheath was inserted. A 6F multipurpose catheter (MPA2) and guide wire were advanced as one unit into inferior vena cava through the sheath; and then into right atrium, ventricle and left pulmonary through the pulmonary valve under echocardiographic guidance. After measuring the right ventricle and pulmonary artery pressure, the guide wire was withdrawn and a super-stiff guide wire was insert, and a BALT balloon with 18 mm in diameter was advanced along the guide wire. The balloon was rapidly inflated with saline for 5 s and reflated for 2 times. After valvuloplasty, the transvalvular gradient was

reduced to 12 mmHg and the oxygen saturation was 100%, which indicated that the pulmonary stenosis was significantly relieved. After procedure, echocardiography examination revealed that the transvalvular pressure gradient was 10 mmHg, and there was mild pulmonary valve regurgitation. ECG and blood test were normal. Antibiotics were given intravenously for 2 days.

Case 2 Patient was 14 years old, female, weight 78 kg (Video 10.2).

The heart murmur was found when she was born. She was developed well. Echocardiographic findings: severe pulmonary valve stenosis, transvalvular pressure gradient was 71 mmHg, mild funnel myocardium hypertrophy. The diameter of pulmonary valve annulus was 19.5 mm. Due to the patient's echocardiographic window was poor, the transesophageal echocardiography was performed for guidance of valvuloplasty procedure. The right femoral vein was punctured, a 11F sheath was placed, and a 6F multipurpose catheter (MPA2) and guide wire were advanced through the arterial sheath into the left pulmonary artery through the pulmonary valve under transesophageal echocardiography guidance. After measuring the right ventricle and pulmonary artery pressure, the guide wire was exchanged to a super-stiff guide wire. A 28 mm BALT balloon catheter was advanced along the guide wire. The balloon was rapidly inflated with saline for 5 s and reflated for 2 times. The pressure gradient between funnel and right ventricle was 34 mmHg, and the transvalvular pressure gradient was 29 mmHg; which indicate that the pulmonary valve stenosis was significantly improved. After procedure, echocardiography examination revealed that the transvalvular pressure gradient was 26 mmHg, and there was mild pulmonary valve regurgitation. ECG and blood test were normal. Antibiotics were given intravenously for 2 days.

Case 3 Patient is 5 years old, male, weighing 18 kg (Video 10.3).

Heart murmur was found more than 1 week ago. He has no history of lip cyanosis, syncope, swelling, or hemoptysis. He is developed well. Echocardiographic findings: severe pulmonary valve stenosis, transvalvular pressure gradient was 72 mmHg, the diameter of pulmonary valve annulus was 14 mm. The pulmonary valvuloplasty was performed under transthoracic echocardiography. The right femoral vein was punctured with a 9F arterial sheath. A 6F right coronary artery catheter and guide wire were advanced as an unit through the arterial sheath and is sent into the left pulmonary artery through the pulmonary valve under echocardiography guidance. After measuring the right ventricle and pulmonary artery pressure through the catheter, the guide wire was exchanged to a super-stiff guide wire. A 20 mm BALT balloon catheter was advanced along the super-stiff guide wire. The balloon was rapidly inflated with saline for 5 s. After valvuloplasty, the pressure gradient between the pulmonary artery and the right ventricle (funnel) was reduced to 9 mmHg, the transvalve gradient was 13 mmHg, and the oxygen saturation was 100%, which indicated that the pulmonary valve stenosis was relieved.

Post-procedure echocardiography examination showed that transvalvular pressure gradient was 12 mmHg. There was no pulmonary valve regurgitation. ECG and blood test were normal. Antibiotics were given intravenously for 2 days.

References

1. Taggart NW, et al. Outcomes for balloon pulmonary valvuloplasty in adults: comparison with a concurrent pediatric cohort. Catheter Cardiovasc Interv. 2013;82(5):811–5.
2. Wang SZ, et al. First-in-human percutaneous balloon valvuloplasty under echocardiographic guidance only. Congenit Heart Dis. 2016;11(6):716–20.
3. Pan XB, H SS, Ouyang WB, et al. Application of percutaneous balloon pulmonary valvuloplasty under echocardiographic guidance. Chin J Pediatr Surg. 2015;36(4):286–8.
4. Rao PS. Percutaneous balloon pulmonary valvuloplasty: state of the art. Catheter Cardiovasc Interv. 2007;69(5):747–63.
5. McCrindle BW. Independent predictors of long-term results after balloon pulmonary valvuloplasty. Valvuloplasty and angioplasty of congenital anomalies (VACA) registry investigators. Circulation. 1994;89(4):1751–9.
6. Harrild DM, et al. Long-term pulmonary regurgitation following balloon valvuloplasty for pulmonary stenosis risk factors and relationship to exercise capacity and ventricular volume and function. J Am Coll Cardiol. 2010;55(10):1041–7.

Echocardiography-Guided Percutaneous Interventions for Aortic Valve Stenosis

11

There are three primary causes of aortic valvular stenosis (AS): rheumatic aortic valve disease, congenital malformation of aortic valve, and degenerative aortic valve disease. Congenital aortic valve dysplasia commonly underlies aortic stenosis in young patients, with bicuspid aortic valve being the most frequent form. Degenerative aortic valve disease is usually seen in patients aged over 65, accounting for over 70% of AS cases among patients aged over 70. Aortic valve disease caused by rheumatic fever is also one of the common causes. The thickening of the leaflets and the fusion of the leaflets and commissures eventually lead to calcification, resulting in narrowing of the valve orifice. This chapter introduces how to do PAN procedure for aortic valve stenosis.

11.1 Anatomy

There are three anatomic forms of valvular AS according to the etiology:

Congenital aortic stenosis: Congenital leaflet malformation (usually bicuspid valve) results in a reduced aortic orifice area, leading to severe calcification after decades. Massive calcific nodules located in leaflet tissue and commissures of the valve, which may also be found in aortic annulus and aortic walls, can cause aortic valve insufficiency.

Rheumatic aortic stenosis: In the early stage, it manifests as limited thickening of the three leaflets and fusion of the commissures, and later with severe calcification of the leaflets and fixed stenosis of the aortic valve.

Degenerative aortic stenosis: The three leaflets structure is often maintained without commissure fusion, and scattered calcification of the valve leaflets leading to fixation of aortic valve orifice can be seen.

11.2 Pathophysiology

Usually, aortic valve orifice area is 3–4 cm^2, and there will be an obvious hemodynamic change when it is reduced to one-fourth of its normal value. Aortic stenosis interferes with left ventricular blood ejection. While severe congenital aortic stenosis may cause early death without timely operation, aortic stenosis in adults evolves slowly and results in compensatory left ventricular hypertrophy, reduced ventricular compliance, diastolic dysfunction, lack and unbalanced distribution of coronary blood flow, and endomyocardial ischemia. The latter damage leads to left ventricular dysfunction in a vicious cycle. Interference with left ventricular blood ejection may result in increased left atrial and pulmonary venous pressure, pulmonary congestion, and exertional dyspnea [1].

11.3 Indications and Contraindications

11.3.1 Indications

The indications usually considered for a procedure are:

(a) Aortic valvuloplasty is indicated regardless of valve gradient in the newborn with isolated critical valvar AS who is ductal dependent or in children with isolated valvar AS who have depressed left ventricular systolic function.

(b) Aortic valvuloplasty is indicated in children with isolated valvar AS who have a resting peak systolic valve gradient (by catheter) of >50 mmHg.

(c) Aortic valvuloplasty is indicated in children with isolated valvar AS who have a resting peak systolic valve gradient (by catheter) of >40 mmHg if there are symptoms of angina or syncope or ischemic ST-T-wave changes on electrocardiography at rest or with exercise.

Electronic Supplementary Material The online version of this chapter (https://doi.org/10.1007/978-981-15-2055-6_11) contains supplementary material, which is available to authorized users.

X. Pan et al., *Percutaneous and Non-fluoroscopical (PAN) Procedure for Structural Heart Disease*, https://doi.org/10.1007/978-981-15-2055-6_11

(d) Aortic valvuloplasty may be considered in a child or adolescent with a resting peak systolic valve gradient (by catheter) of >40 mmHg but without symptoms or ST–T-wave changes if the patient desires to become pregnant or to participate in strenuous competitive sports [2].

(e) Aortic valvuloplasty may be considered for asymptomatic patients with a catheter-obtained peak systolic gradient of <50 mmHg when the patient is heavily sedated or anesthetized if a nonsedated Doppler study finds the mean valve gradient to be >50 mmHg [3].

11.3.2 Contraindications

The following clinical situations are usually considered as contraindications:

(a) Asymptomatic patient with aortic stenosis, normal left ventricular function and invasive peak-to-peak systolic transaortic valve gradient <40 mmHg, without ECG change

(b) Patient with aortic stenosis combined with moderate regurgitation

(c) When aortic replacement or repair is necessary

(d) In the presence of thrombus or infective endocarditis

11.4 Preoperative Examination

Routine laboratory and imaging evaluation are needed and include: echocardiogram, chest X-ray, the electrocardiogram, and routine hematological and biochemistry tests.

Additional tests for myocardial enzyme levels and pulmonary function, and Holter monitor should be performed if needed.

Preoperative transthoracic echocardiography should focus on the following data: LV function; evaluation of aortic valve morphology, function, annular and valve size, systolic maximum, and mean aortic valve gradient. Furthermore, the presence of associated defects should be taken into consideration;

Informed and signed consent should be obtained from parents in case of children. In older patients and adults, the patient should sign too.

11.5 Procedure

The patient is placed in a supine position under general anesthesia and tracheal intubation. Echocardiography is performed before the procedure to measure the aortic annulus diameter and maximal peak and mean systolic transaortic valve gradient (Fig. 11.1). In our experience, a 6F arterial sheath is inserted into right internal jugular vein, and the temporary pacing lead is advanced to the right ventricle. A temporary external pacemaker is connected for backup and in case of need for overdrive pacing in order to stabilize balloon position.

The right femoral arterial access is obtained by using a sheath compatible with patient age and aortic annulus size (that will take account of the balloon chosen for the balloon angioplasty). A 5 or 6 Fr multipurpose catheter (MPA2) and a guide wire (PTFE-coated super stiff straight tip, Cordis, 260 cm, 035 in.) are advanced from the arterial access. Aortic pressure in the ascending aorta is recorded. By using a long-

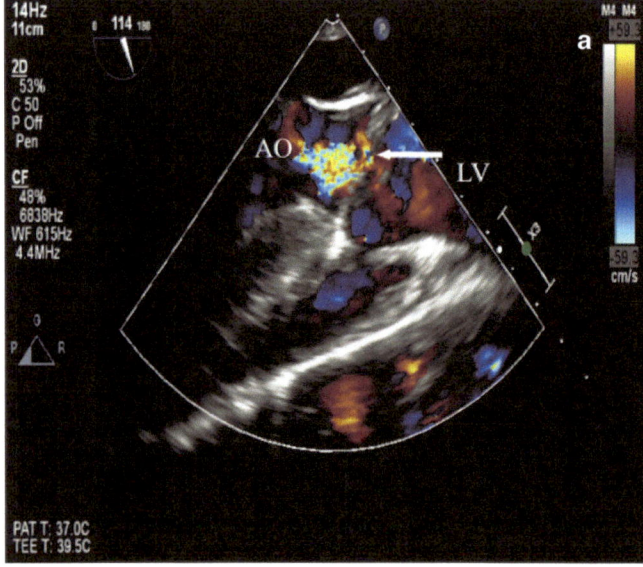
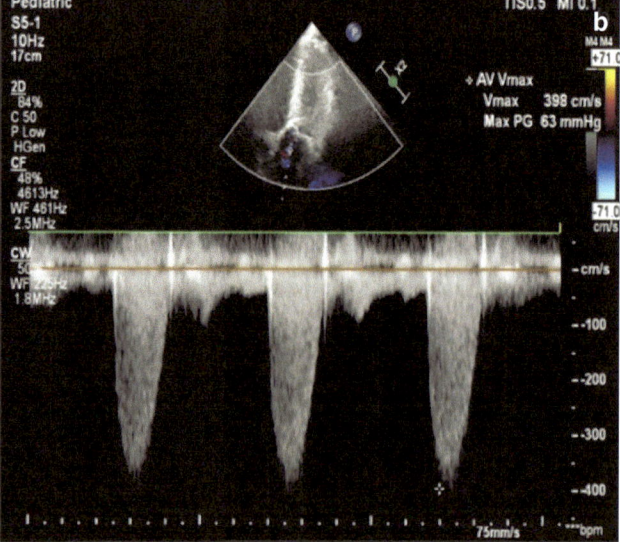

Fig. 11.1 Transesophageal echocardiography before procedure: (**a**) Color Doppler showed high velocity of transaortic blood flow (↑). (**b**) Continuous wave Doppler recording shows a maximal systolic gradient of 63 mmHg

axis view of the aorta under echocardiography surveillance, the catheter and the guide wire position are adjusted appropriately. Repeated gentle attempts to advance the guide wire through the aortic valve into the left ventricle might be needed. Sometimes, a right Judkins coronary artery catheter may be helpful to advance the guide wire across the aortic valve. After measuring the pressure of the left ventricle through the catheter, an exchange super-stiff guide wire is advanced. Then, before withdrawing the catheter, we mark the depth of catheter itself as working length.

A BALT balloon (BALT, France, 20 mm) is advanced along the guide wire, and the diameter of the balloon is chosen not to exceed the diameter of the aortic annulus. When the insertion depth of the balloon catheter reaches the working length, the balloon can be partially inflated to adjust the position of the balloon so that the middle portion of the balloon is located at the aortic annulus under echocardiography guidance.

With temporary rapid pacing, the balloon catheter and guide wire are fixed, and the balloon is rapidly inflated to expand the aortic valve (Fig. 11.2). After dilatation, the balloon is deflated and retracted into the aorta. The aortic valve orifice area, gradient, and regurgitation can be analyzed by echocardiography (Fig. 11.3). If the results were not satisfactory, the balloon diameter should be increased and a new

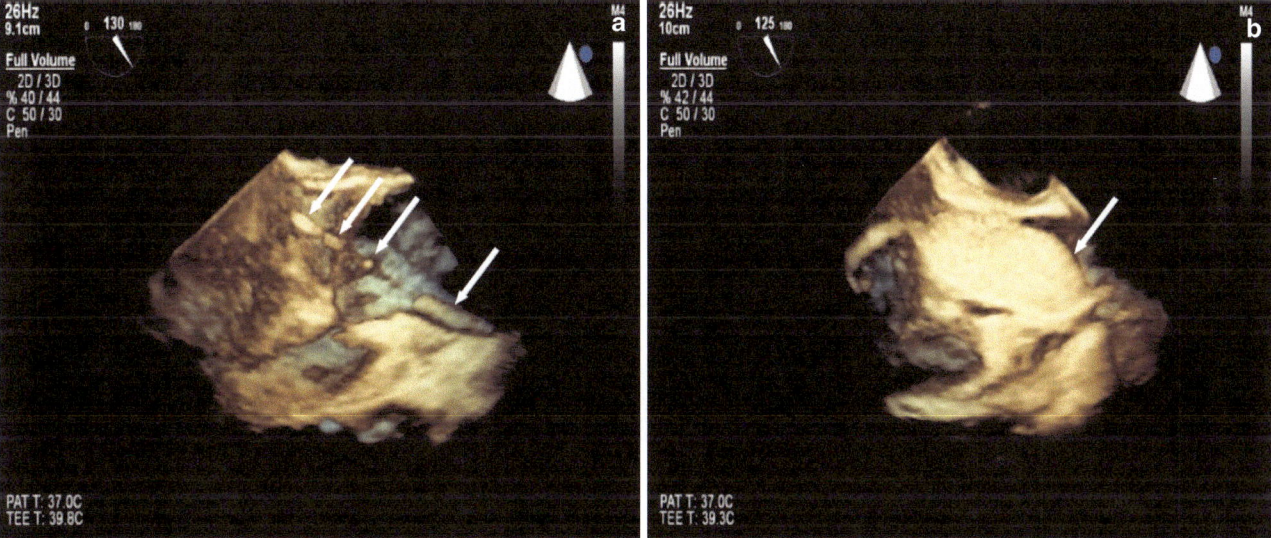

Fig. 11.2 Three-dimensional (3D) echocardiography: (**a**) Balloon catheter (↑) passes through the aortic valve. (**b**) The balloon (↑) is inflated with microbubble saline

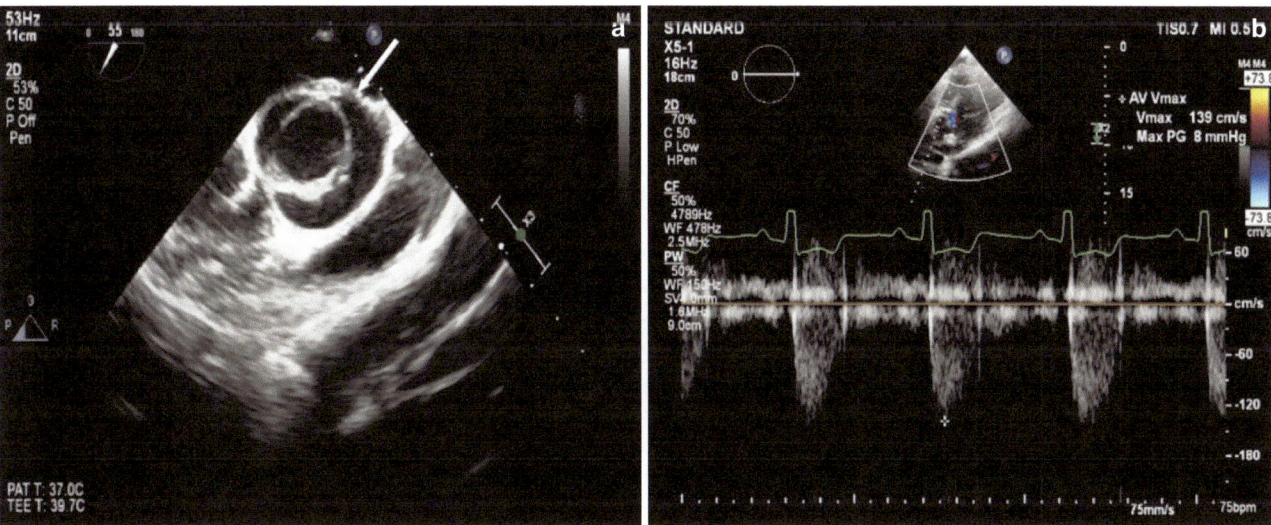

Fig. 11.3 Transesophageal echocardiography after valvuloplasty: (**a**) The aortic valve orifice area (↑) is increased. (**b**) The transaortic gradient is significantly decreased

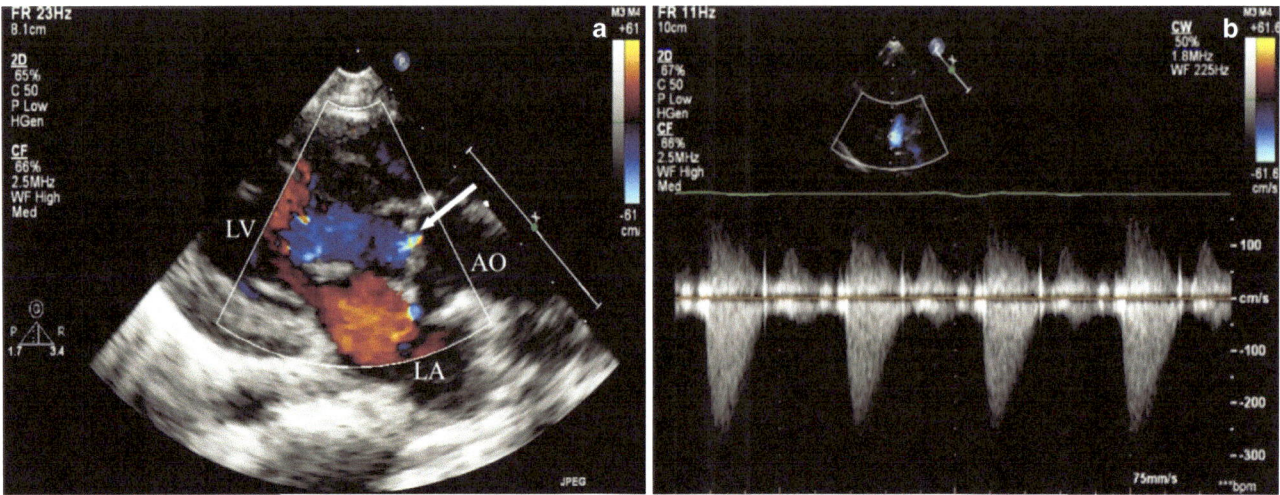

Fig. 11.4 Transthoracic echocardiography before procedure: (**a**) Parasternal long-axis view shows the limitation of aortic valve (↑) motion; (**b**) Continuous wave Doppler recording for measuring transaortic gradient

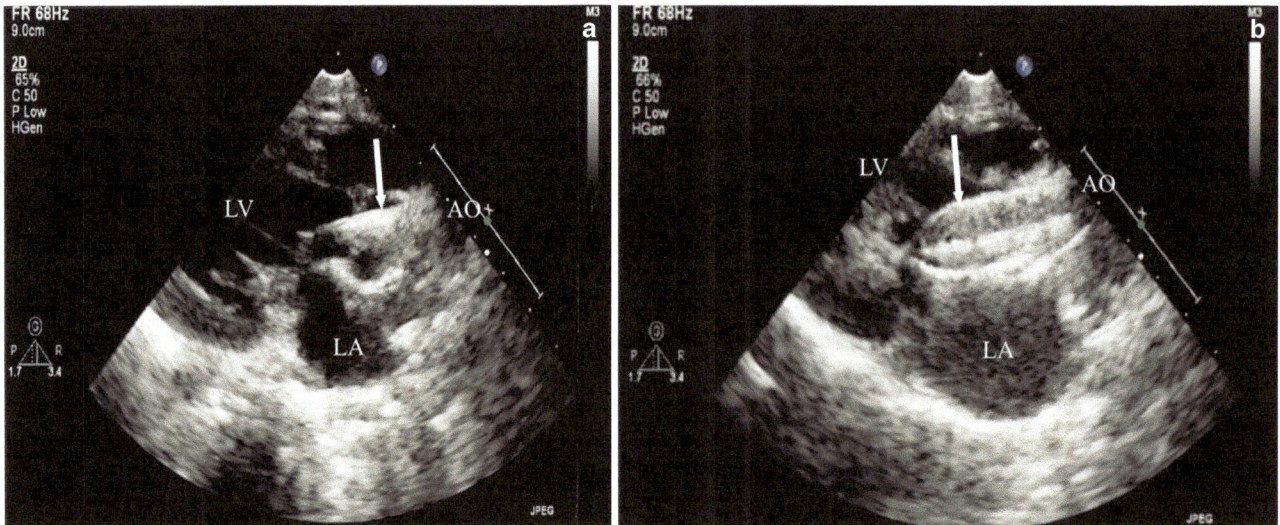

Fig. 11.5 Transthoracic echocardiography: (**a**) Parasternal long-axis view shows the balloon (↑) catheter has passed the aortic valve. (**b**) Same view shows the balloon is inflated with microbubble saline

angioplasty could be performed. After satisfactory dilation is obtained, the catheter, the guide wire, and the arterial sheath are withdrawn [4–6]. Manual groin compression is performed to stop bleeding, and a compressive bandage is placed. The transthoracic echocardiography-guiding procedure is shown in Figs. 11.4, 11.5, and 11.6.

11.6 Postoperative Care

After the procedure patients should rest in bed for 12 h. The ECG, vital signs, including heart rate, heart rhythm, blood pressure, oxygen saturation, should be monitored for 24 h. The puncture site and the pulsation of the dorsal artery of the foot should be observed to find hematoma and the isch-

emia caused by the compression puncture point in time. Antibiotics are given intravenously once half an hour pre-procedure and 6 h post-procedure. Echocardiographic examination should be performed within 24 h, 1, 3, 6, and 12 months post-procedure and every other year thereafter.

11.7 Postoperative Complications and Treatment

1. Aortic valve regurgitation. According to literature report, the incidence of moderate-to-severe aortic regurgitation is 4%, which can cause acute left heart failure and requires valve surgical replacement. But in most cases, regurgitation after valvuloplasty is mild. This complication is cur-

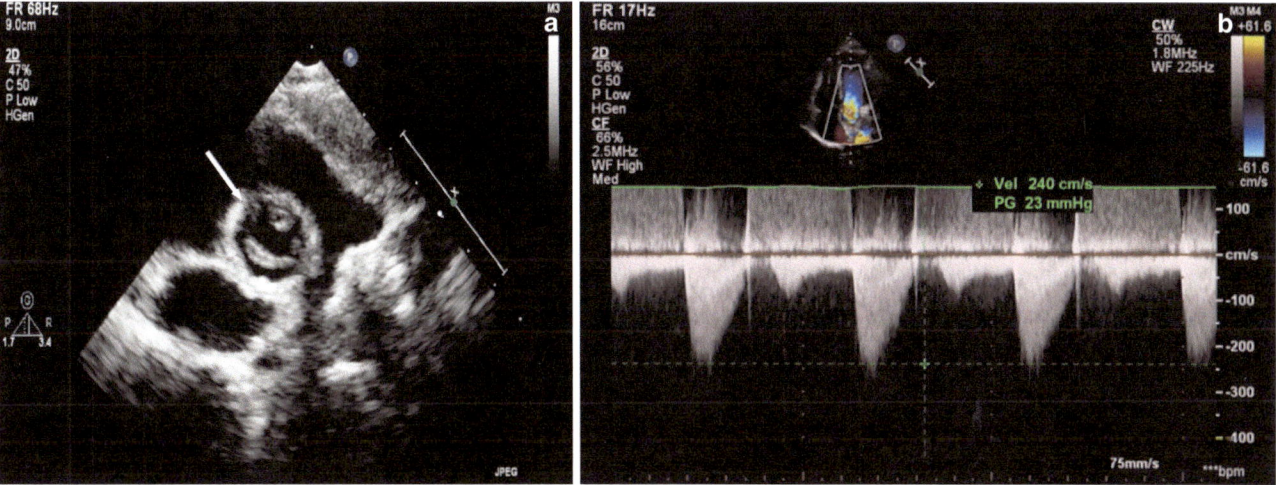

Fig. 11.6 Transthoracic echocardiography after valvuloplasty: (**a**) The aortic valve orifice area (↑) is increased. (**b**) The transaortic gradient is significantly decreased

rently considered to be related to the balloon/valve ratio being too large; therefore, the diameter of the balloon should not exceed the diameter of the aortic annulus to avoid a moderate-to-severe aortic valve regurgitation.

2. Femoral artery thrombosis or vascular injury. Femoral artery injury may occur in 12% of valvuloplasty. The medical treatment of thrombosis includes thrombolytic therapy such as heparin and urokinase; surgical treatment includes local thrombectomy and vascular injury repair.

3. Arrhythmia. Arrhythmias are common in PBAV, and transient electrocardiographic abnormalities often occur. Rapid arrhythmias include premature beats, supraventricular tachycardia, ventricular tachycardia, and even ventricular fibrillation. Most of the above arrhythmias are transient. They are usually related to catheter and wires manipulation within the heart. When severe arrhythmias occur, then an urgent treatment is needed. It includes withdrawal of the balloon catheter, drugs infusion, external electric shock, and pacemaker adjuvant therapy.

4. Embolization. Small blood clots, air, or detached valve fragments can cause embolization in arterial system during catheter procedure. Therefore, heparin needs to be injected at a dose of 80–100 U/kg of heparin in order to keep an ACT >250 s during the procedure. The balloon catheter should be carefully deflated and retracted so that even if a balloon rupture occurs during inflation, it will not cause air embolism [7, 8].

11.8 Advantages of Echocardiography Guidance

Echocardiography guidance has a clear advantage over radiation guidance in assessing cardiac structure and hemodynamic. Firstly, the catheter guide wire can be adjusted according to the direction of blood flow under guidance of echocardiography, making it easier to pass through the stenotic aortic valve. Secondly, the correct position of the balloon can be checked in real time under guidance of echocardiography. The position of balloon is not clearly visible under X-ray, and the balloon can easily slip during the inflation process, leading to failure in achieving an effective valvuloplasty. Finally, the results, such as valvular regurgitation, and the occurrence of pericardial effusion may be better estimated by echocardiography in real time [5, 8].

11.9 Case (Video 11.1)

Case 1 Patient is a 45 years old, female, height 176 cm, weight 69 kg (Video 11.1) who was admitted due to palpitations, dizziness, and fatigue.

Physical examination: Heart rate was 95 beats/min, blood pressure was 106/79 mmHg, blood oxygen saturation was 98%, and heart rhythm was normal. A 3–4/6 systolic murmur was heard at aortic valve area. Echocardiography showed that the left and right coronary leaflets of aortic valve were fused as bicuspid aortic valve; furthermore, the aortic leaflets were slightly thickened. The maximal systolic peak transaortic gradient was 63 mmHg, the diameter of aortic valve annulus was 23 mm. The ascending aorta showed post-stenotic dilatation. The final diagnosis was bicuspid aortic valve with severe aortic stenosis. Therefore, a percutaneous balloon aortic valvuloplasty was recommended.

Procedure: The patient was placed in supine position with general anesthesia, and tracheal intubation. The echocardiography examination was performed before procedure to measure the diameter of aortic annulus and aortic valve gradient. A right internal jugular vein was obtained and a 6F arterial sheath was inserted. A temporary pacing lead was placed into the right ventricle and connected to an external temporary pacemaker. The right femoral artery was punctured, and a 10F sheath was placed. The 6F multipurpose catheter (MPA2) and super-stiff guide wire were advanced through the sheath. The catheter and guide wire crossed the aortic valve into the left ventricle under echocardiography guidance. The super-stiff guide wire was exchanged and a 20 mm BALT balloon (BALT, France) was advanced along the guide wire. After the balloon catheter insertion reached the working length, the balloon was partially inflated, and the position of the balloon was adjusted to put the middle portion of the balloon at the aortic annulus under echocardiography guidance. Under temporary rapid pacing (heart rate 180–200 beats/min), the balloon catheter and guide wire were fixed, and the balloon was rapidly inflated to expand the aortic valve. The aortic valvuloplasty was performed twice with a 20 mm × 3 cm and 23 mm × 4.5 cm balloon, respectively. After valvuloplasty, the balloon was deflated and retracted into the aorta. The aortic valvular function was estimated by 2D and Doppler echocardiography to ensure the aortic valvular function was well without severe regurgitation. If the result was satisfactory, the catheter, the guide wire, and the sheath were withdrawn. Manual compression of the puncture site was performed.

Outcome: The patient's symptoms significantly improved. The maximal systolic transaortic gradient was reduced from 63 to 14 mmHg after procedure. The aortic valve orifice area was increased from 0.9 to 2.0 cm^2. The procedure time was 30 min; the intraoperative blood loss was 20 mL. The patient was discharged 2 days after procedure. At follow-up, the patient is doing well.

References

1. Feldman T. Balloon aortic valvuloplasty: still under-developed after two decades of use. Catheter Cardiovasc Interv. 2013;81(2):374–5.
2. Elkayam U, Bitar F. Valvular heart disease and pregnancy part I: native valves. J Am Coll Cardiol. 2005;46(2):223–30.
3. Khawaja MZ, et al. Standalone balloon aortic valvuloplasty: indications and outcomes from the UK in the transcatheter valve era. Catheter Cardiovasc Interv. 2013;81(2):366–73.
4. Pan XB, Pang KJ, Hu SS, et al. Safety and efficacy of percutaneous transcatheter closure of atrial septal defect under transesophageal echocardiography guidance in children. Chin J Cardiol. 2013;41(9):744–6.
5. Bourgault C, et al. Usefulness of Doppler echocardiography guidance during balloon aortic valvuloplasty for the treatment of congenital aortic stenosis. Int J Cardiol. 2008;128(1):30–7.
6. Ben-Dor I, et al. Balloon aortic valvuloplasty for severe aortic stenosis as a bridge to transcatheter/surgical aortic valve replacement. Catheter Cardiovasc Interv. 2013;82(4):632–7.
7. Meinel FG, et al. Radiation risks from cardiovascular imaging tests. Circulation. 2014;130(5):442–5.
8. Baysson H, et al. Risk of cancer associated with cardiac catheterization procedures during childhood: a cohort study in France. BMC Public Health. 2013;13:266.

Mitral stenosis (MS) is more common in women, with a male: female ratio from 2:3 to 3:4. Rheumatic fever is the most important cause of mitral stenosis [1], accounting for 80–90% of mitral stenosis. Other possible causes include infective endocarditis, mitral annular calcification (MAC), cardiac tumors, endomyocardial fibrosis (EMF), etc. Approximately, 25–40% of all patients with rheumatic heart disease have pure MS. This chapter introduces how to perform PAN procedure for mitral stenosis.

12.1 Anatomical Features

The inflammation caused by rheumatic fever may lead to edema and fibrinous exudation of mitral valve leaflet and further calcification and fibrosis in the components of mitral valve apparatus, leading to mitral valve stenosis. According to the degree of lesions, mitral stenosis can be divided into four types:

1. Membranous stenosis: Thickening and adhesion only at the edge of leaflets. The leaflet lesion is slight without restricted leaflet mobility.
2. Membrane thickening type: Membranous stenosis with thickening leaflets. The leaflet mobility is partially restricted and tendinous cords are slightly fused.
3. Membrane funnel type: The leaflets thicken and become rigid, whereas the chords can be shortened and fused. The leaflet is pulled down like a restricted funnel. The leaflet mobility is restricted with mitral insufficiency.
4. Funnel shape: The leaflet thickens; the tendinous cords and papillary muscles are obviously fibrotic shortened and fused. The orifice is funnel-shaped and the leaflet mobility is obviously restricted, accompanied by mitral insufficiency.

Electronic Supplementary Material The online version of this chapter (https://doi.org/10.1007/978-981-15-2055-6_12) contains supplementary material, which is available to authorized users.

12.2 Pathophysiology

The mitral valve orifice area of normal adult is 4–6 cm^2. When the orifice area of the mitral valve is less than 2 cm^2, the hemodynamic will change significantly. Blood flow from the left atrium to the left ventricle is blocked, and the left atrial pressure is increased. The pressure gradient between the left atrium and the left ventricle must be increased to maintain blood flow. When the mitral valve orifice area is less than 1 cm^2, the left atrial-left ventricular pressure gradient has exceeded 20 mmHg, and pulmonary vein and pulmonary capillary pressures are significantly increased, resulting in pulmonary congestion. When the patient is tired or emotional, the blood volume of the pulmonary veins and pulmonary capillaries is significantly increased, and symptoms such as exertional dyspnea and hemoptysis may occur. Severe pulmonary congestion can lead to pulmonary spasm, passive increase in pulmonary arterial pressure, and long-term pulmonary arteriosclerosis, stenosis, and eventually develop into severe pulmonary hypertension. When the pulmonary artery pressure exceeds 60 mmHg, right ventricular emptying is severely blocked, which can lead to right heart failure [2].

12.3 Indications and Contraindications

12.3.1 Indications

1. Patients with moderate and severe simple mitral stenosis, fusion at the junction, good leaflet activity, no calcification, mild fusion or hypertrophy of mitral apparatus, no mitral regurgitation, no thrombus in the left atrium, sinus rhythm, echocardiographic Wilkins score ≤8 points (Table 12.1).
2. Patients with severe mitral stenosis have surgical contraindications or surgically high risk.
3. Patients have pulmonary hypertension (systolic pressure >50 mmHg at rest), but require major noncardiac surgery or have pregnancy requirements [3, 4].

X. Pan et al., *Percutaneous and Non-fluoroscopical (PAN) Procedure for Structural Heart Disease*,
https://doi.org/10.1007/978-981-15-2055-6_12

Table 12.1 Wilkins score

Grade	Mobility	Thickening	Calcification	Subvalvular thickening
1	Highly mobile with only leaflet tips restricted	Leaflets near normal in thickness (4–5 mm)	A single area of increased echo brightness	Minimal thickening just below the mitral leaflets
2	Leaflet mid portions and base portions have normal mobility	Mid-leaflets normal, considerable thickening of margins (5–8 mm)	Scattered areas of brightness confined to leaflet margins	Thickening of chordal structures extending to one of the chordal length
3	Valve continues to move forward in diastole, mainly from the base	Thickening extending through the entire leaflets (5–8 mm)	Brightness extending into the mid portions of the leaflets	Thickening extended to distal third of chords
4	No or minimal forward movement of the leaflets in diastole	Considerable thickening of all leaflet tissue (>8–10 mm)	Extensive brightness throughout much of the leaflet tissue	Extensive thickening and shortening of all chordal structures extending down to the papillary muscle

Fig. 12.1 Device of mitral valvuloplasty

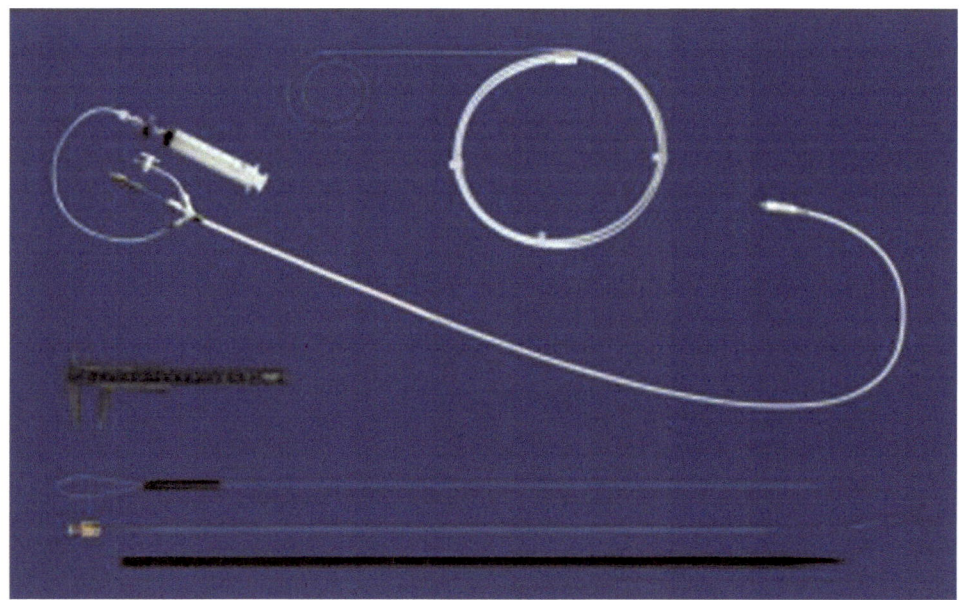

12.3.2 Contraindications

During the rheumatic activity period, there is a history of systemic embolism and severe arrhythmia. The valve leaflets are severely deformed and curled, and the subvalvular structure is severely fused. There are moderate-to-severe mitral valvular regurgitation.

12.4 Preoperative Preparation

1. Routine laboratory and imaging examination: Including chest X-ray, electrocardiogram, echocardiography, blood routine, hepatic and renal function and blood electrolytes, coagulation time and indicators of infectious disease. The purpose of the examination is to comprehensively evaluate the cardiac, hepatic, and renal function for the patients. Patients with persistent atrial fibrillation should have a chest CT scan to assess left atrial thrombosis.
2. Preoperative transthoracic (TTE) and/or transesophageal echocardiography (TEE) examinations focused on the following: evaluation of mitral valve morphology,

function, mitral valve orifice size, and the presence of thrombus in the left atrium. For patients with atrial fibrillation or clinically suspected left atrial thrombus, transesophageal echocardiography should be performed before surgery to exclude the left atrial thrombus.
3. Sign the surgical informed consent before surgery to inform the relevant risks and possible complications.

12.5 Procedure

12.5.1 Device Preparation

1. 16G percutaneous needle, 14F femoral vascular sheath, 6F MPA2 catheter, cook super-stiff guide wire (260 cm), 71 cm atrial septal puncture needle and 8F SR0 puncture sheath (Mullins sheath), Inoue mitral balloon expansion device, and pressure monitoring device (Fig. 12.1). Balloon size (mm) = height (cm)/10 + 10.
2. Anesthesia: The patient is placed in the supine position. Transthoracic echocardiography is performed before the operation to confirm mitral valve orifice and transvalvular

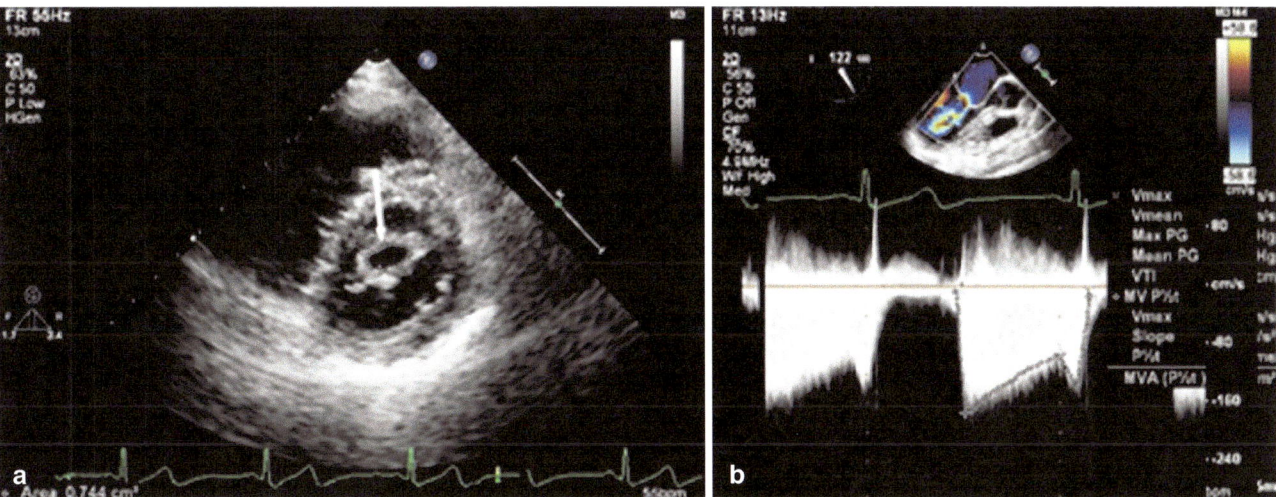

Fig. 12.2 (**a**) Transthoracic echocardiogram: parasternal short-axis view shows mitral valve orifice (↑). (**b**) Transesophageal Doppler recording shows trans-mitral valve gradient

pressure gradient (Fig. 12.2). According to the patient's transthoracic acoustic view, determine whether it is necessary to use transesophageal echocardiography. Transesophageal echocardiography guidance generally requires general anesthesia, tracheal intubation. Under transthoracic echocardiography guidance, anesthesia can be accomplished by local infiltration of 1% lidocaine in the right inguinal region.

3. Femoral vein puncture: After satisfactory anesthesia is administered, 16G percutaneous needle is used to puncture the right femoral vein. The distance from the right parasternal third intercostal space to the puncture site is measured and marked as the first working length. The 14F femoral vascular sheath is placed through the right femoral vein.

4. Trans-septal puncture: A 6F MPA2 catheter and guide wire are advanced through the sheath. The catheter insertion length is consistent with the first working length. The multipurpose catheter (MPA2) is advanced to the atrial septum near the fossa ovalis under echocardiogram guidance. The multipurpose catheter (MPA2) withdrawn, the guide wire is retained in the right atrium, and the Mullins sheath is delivered along the guide wire under echocardiography guidance. The sheath insertion length is the same as the length of the MPA2 catheter was inserted into the body, the guide wire is withdrawn. The Brockenbrough needle is passed through the Mullins sheath, and the needle tail is kept 1 cm outside the sheath under the guidance of echocardiography. The position of the Mullins sheath is adjusted to be placed on the interatrial septum, and the echocardiographic image can be seen as a tent-like deformation. Adjust the position of the puncture site by rotating and pushing the Mullins sheath (Fig. 12.3). The location of Brockenbrough needle tip should be reconfirmed by four-chamber, double-chamber, aortic short-axis views of echocardiography. The operator holds the

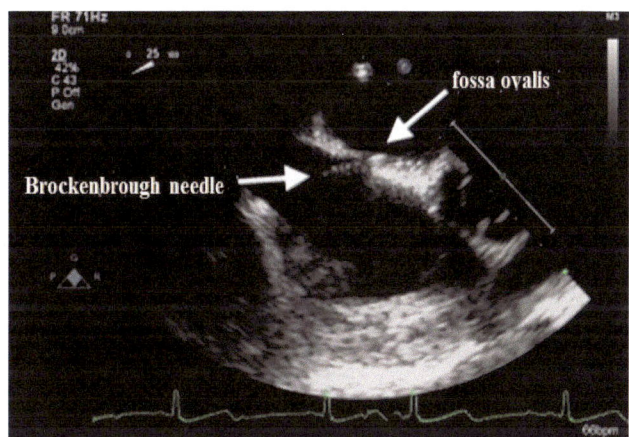

Fig. 12.3 Transesophageal echocardiography: short-axis view shows a Brockenbrough needle (↑) was in the fossa ovalis

puncture sheath and advances the needle to perforate the atrial septum, which has a slight breakthrough feeling. Successful entry into the left atrium should be confirmed by withdrawal of oxygenated blood from the puncture needle. In case of uncertainty, a flush test is useful to confirm adequate access. The ultrasonographical visualization of water bubbles in the left artrium after injection of a small amount of heparin saline via the catheter is used to adequately verify access to the atrial septum (Fig. 12.4).

5. After confirming the successful puncture, hold the puncture needle, gently advance the Mullins sheath into the left atrium, withdraw the puncture needle, record the left atrial pressure, and insert the left atrium guide wire through the sheath. The guide wire is retained, and the Mullins sheath is withdrawn. The correct length of catheter insertion is measured, and defined as the second working length. Heparin is injected via peripheral vein at 80 U/kg, and ACT is monitored and maintained >250 s.

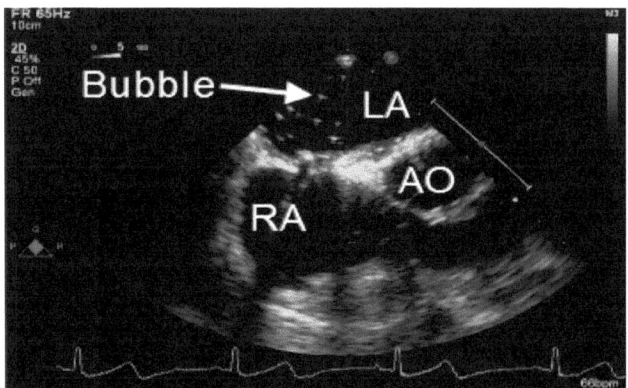

Fig. 12.4 Transesophageal echocardiography: short-axis view shows there was bubbles (↑) in the left atrium

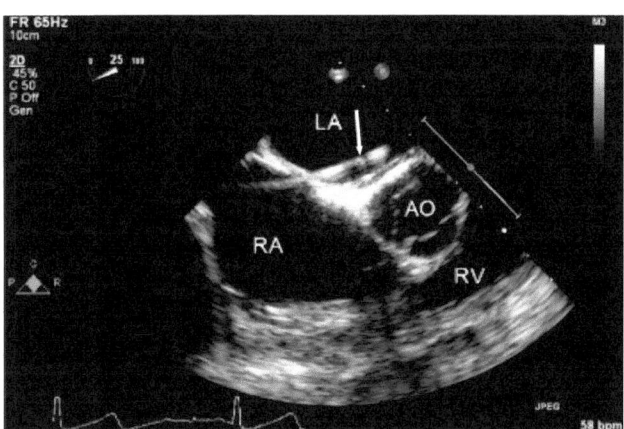

Fig. 12.5 Transesophageal echocardiography: short-axis view shows the balloon catheter (↑) is in the left atrium through atrial septum

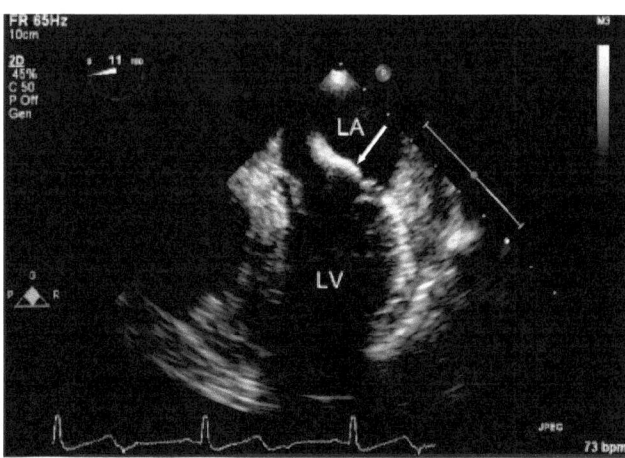

Fig. 12.6 Transesophageal echocardiography shows the balloon catheter (↑) is in the left atrium close to mitral valve orifice

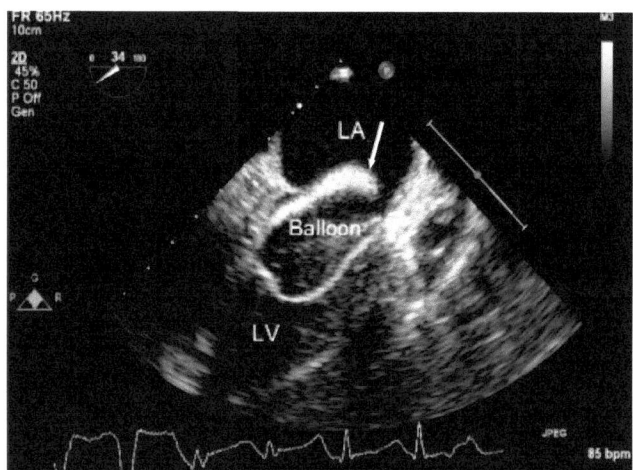

Fig. 12.7 Transesophageal echocardiography shows the balloon (↑) is inflated

6. Balloon catheter operation: The interatrial septum is dilated with a long 14F dilator over the left atrium guide wire. The insertion length is consistent with the second working length. The dilator is removed. An Inoue balloon is passed through the guide wire, with its length exceeding the second working length by 3 cm. The stretching metal tube and left atrium guide wire are removed (Fig. 12.5). A "J" Stylet wire is introduced into the balloon catheter. By maneuvering the balloon catheter while rotating and pushing the Stylet, the balloon tip will move toward the mitral orifice under echocardiography guidance (Fig. 12.6). The balloon can be partially inflated to aid in adjusting the position of the balloon during this procedure. After making sure that the balloon is located at the mitral valve orifice, it is rapidly inflated to dilate the mitral valve (Fig. 12.7). After the waist of the balloon is fully expanded, the fluid in the balloon should be quickly deflated, and the balloon catheter is gently withdrawn to the left atrium. At this time, the balloon can be inflated slightly with a small amount of saline to prevent it dropping into the right atrium.

7. Evaluation of mitral valvuloplasty effect: After dilatation, the balloon is deflated and withdrawn into the left atrium, and the left atrial pressure is measured. The mitral valve orifice area and the degree of mitral regurgitation should be assessed by echocardiography (Fig. 12.8). After successful PBMV, fused commissures are separated, and the mitral valve becomes relatively more mobile. Moreover, the average left atrial pressure is reduced to less than 11 mmHg, the transvalvular pressure gradient is reduced to less than 8 mmHg, and if less than 6 mmHg is superior. The echocardiographic findings indicate that the valve area has increased to >1.5 cm^2, which indicated that the mitral valvuloplasty is successful, and if more than 2 cm^2 is superior. After satisfied expansion, the catheter, the guide wire, and the vascular sheath are withdrawn [5, 6].

8. TTE-guided PBMV: Figs. 12.9, 12.10, 12.11, 12.13, and 12.14.

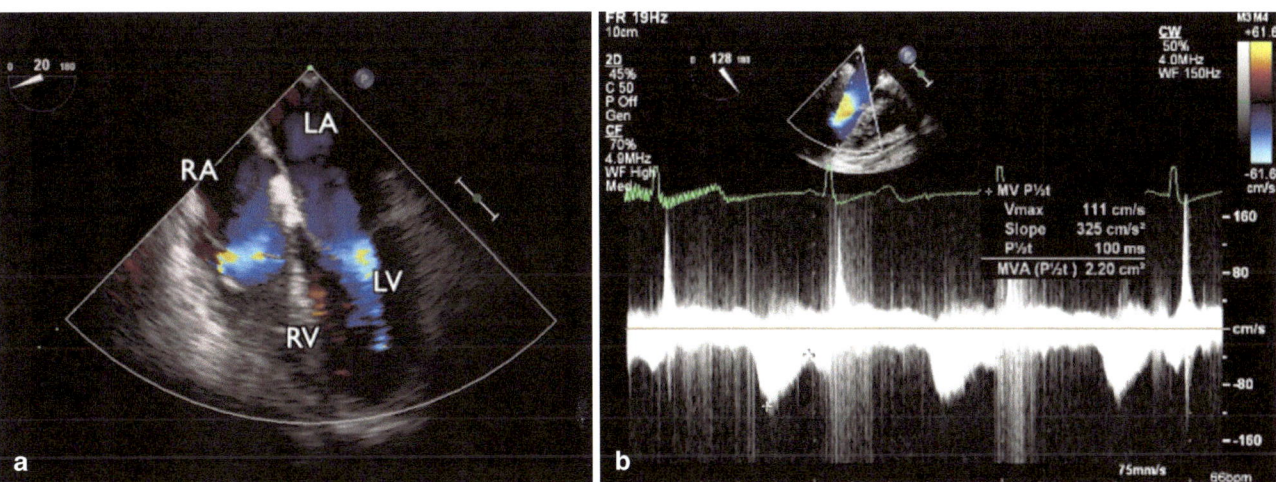

Fig. 12.8 Transesophageal echocardiography after mitral valvuloplasty: (**a**) four-chamber view shows color Doppler recording of mitral valve inflow. (**b**) Transesophageal Doppler recording of mitral valve inflow shows the velocity is decreased

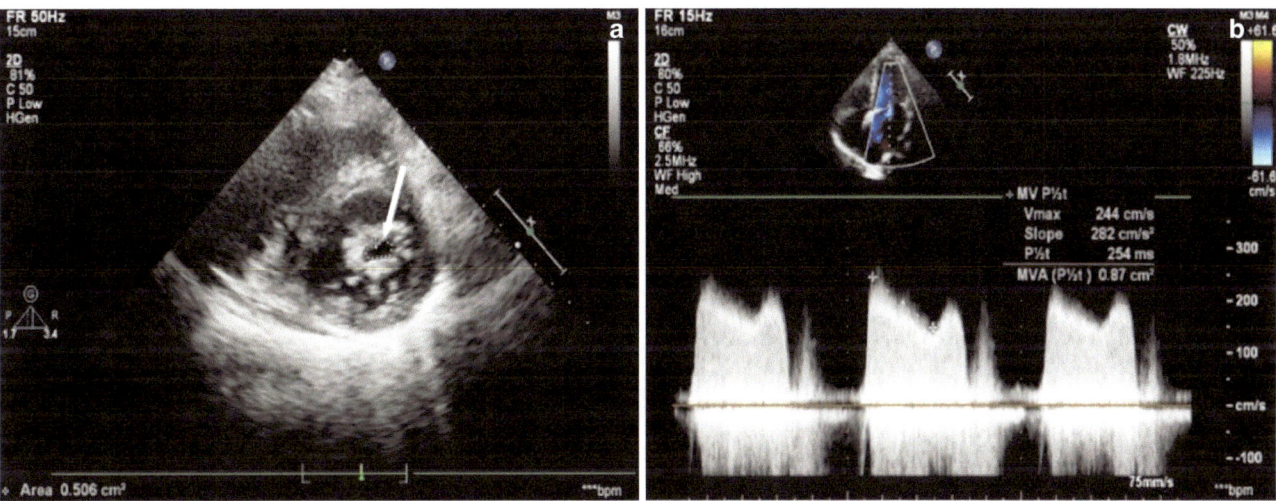

Fig. 12.9 Transthoracic echocardiograph before procedure: (**a**) Two-dimensional parasternal short-axis view at mitral valve level shows the mitral valve orifice (↑). (**b**) The Doppler recording of mitral inflow shows the velocity is high

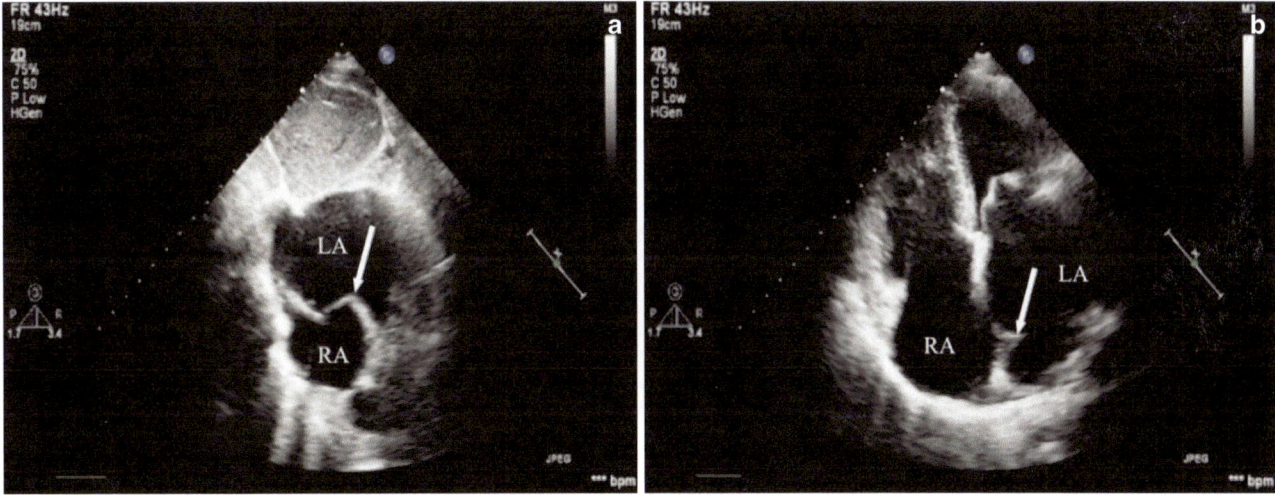

Fig. 12.10 Transthoracic echocardiography: (**a**) Subcostal view shows the fossa ovalis, which is the position of transseptal puncture (↑). (**b**) Apical four-chamber view shows the interseptum is abrupt to left atrial side by a sharp puncture sheath (↑) pushing

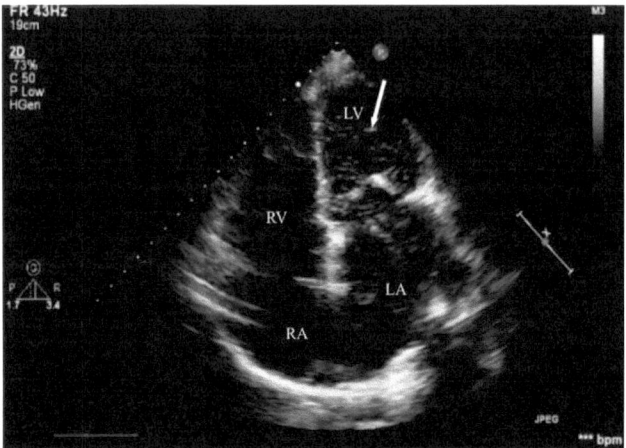

Fig. 12.11 Transthoracic echocardiography: apical four-chamber view shows there were bubbles (↑) in the left atrium and ventricle, which indicated that the transseptal puncture is successful

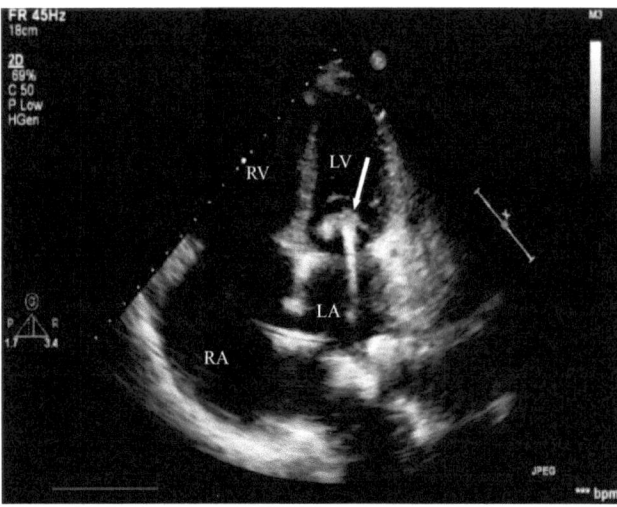

Fig. 12.12 Transthoracic echocardiography: apical four-chamber view shows the balloon catheter (↑) is in the mitral valve orifice

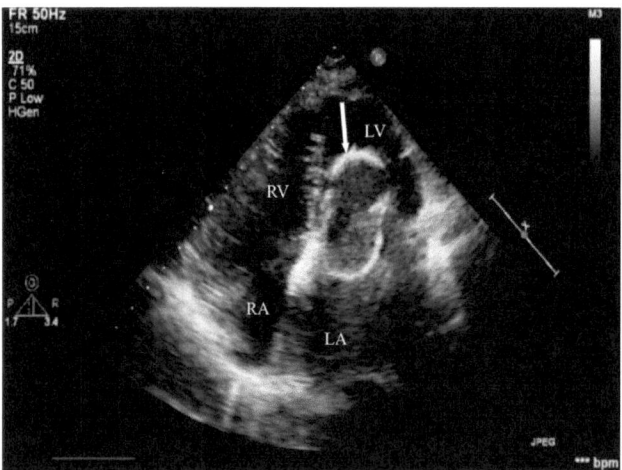

Fig. 12.13 Transthoracic echocardiography: apical four-chamber view shows the balloon catheter (↑) is in the mitral valve orifice and inflated

12.6 Postoperative Care

After procedure, patients should rest in bed for 12 h. The ECG, blood pressure, heart rate, and oxygen saturation should be monitored for 24 h in order to treat timely. And pay attention to observe whether there is hematoma in the puncture site and the pulsation of the dorsal artery of the foot to prevent the lower extremity ischemia caused by the compression of puncture point. Antibiotics are given intravenously once half an hour pre-procedure and 6 h post-procedure. The echocardiography, electrocardiogram, and X-ray chest film should be performed within 24 h after procedure. The patients should be followed up with echocardiographic examination at 1, 3, 6, and 12 months after procedure. Patients with atrial fibrillation are advised to take warfarin anticoagulation for a long time and monitor the international normalized ratio (INR) and maintain an INR between 1.5 and 2.0.

12.7 Postoperative Complications and Treatment

12.7.1 Pericardial Tamponade

Cardiac tamponade after septal puncture is a major complication of mitral valvuloplasty. The incidence rate reported in the literature before 1994 was 1.66–3.66%. In recent years, with the popularization and improvement of this technology, the incidence has decreased to 0.2–2.2%. It is mainly caused by transseptal puncture technique, such as incorrect interatrial puncture site, brockenbrough needle advanced too far, guide wire or catheter injury left atrium or pulmonary veins [2].

Patients with a small amount of pericardial effusion can be observed and continue to receive PBMV treatment. A large amount of pericardial effusion will lead to pericardial tamponade, requiring immediately pericardial puncture drainage or emergency surgical operation.

12.7.2 Severe Mitral Regurgitation

The incidence of this complication is 1.16–12.4%. The main causes include: (1) valve conditions are not optimal. Domestic scholars have suggested that the anterior valve mobility is an important factor in determining whether to cause mitral regurgitation; (2) balloon diameter is too large; (3) too many times of balloon inflations; and (4) incorrect operation, such as inflation of the balloon into the papillary muscles or chordae, leading to rupture of the papillary muscles or chordae. Preventive methods include: (1) Strict indications. Research shows that Wilkins score

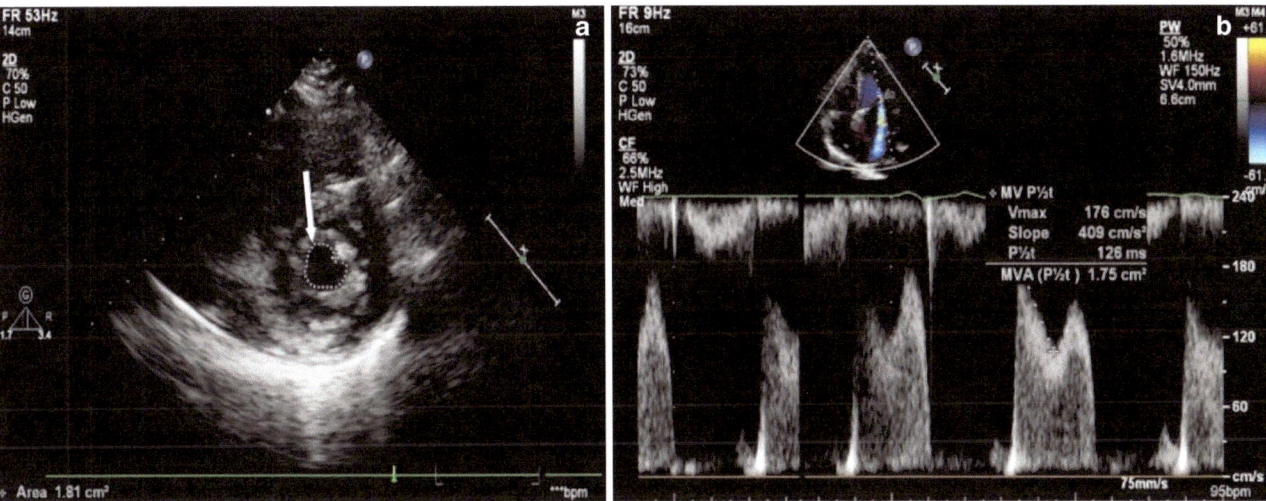

Fig. 12.14 Transthoracic echocardiography after valvuloplasty: (**a**) Parasternal short-axis view at mitral valve level shows the mitral valve orifice (↑). (**b**) Shows Doppler recording of mitral valvular inflow

has certain practical significance in selecting cases for PBMV. (2) Choose the appropriate balloon catheter and inflation diameter. (3) Clear treatment goals: to improve clinical symptoms as the first goal, but not the pursuit of the size of the valve area, especially for patients with unsatisfactory valve conditions. (4) Avoid the balloon catheter entering into the papillary muscles or chordae. In the event of severe mitral regurgitation, diuretic therapy should be aggressively treated. In the case of ineffective conservative treatment, surgical mitral valve replacement is required.

12.7.3 Acute Pulmonary Edema

Common causes include: severe mitral stenosis, high left atrial pressure, intraoperative nervous tension, catheter-induced arrhythmia, and balloon dilation leading to severe MR.

Preventive measures: Complete preoperative preparation, patients with severe cardiac congestion should be treated with diuresis; AF patients with fast ventricular rate should be treated with digoxin and beta-blockers post-PBMV. In addition, the operation time should be shortened as much as possible to avoid the occurrence of severe mitral regurgitation.

12.7.4 Thrombosis and Embolism

Patients with atrial fibrillation have a higher risk of developing thrombosis and embolism, with an incidence of about 1–3%; therefore, they should receive long-term oral warfarin to prevent thrombosis and embolism events.

12.7.5 Restenosis

Because of variation in baseline status of patients undergoing PBMV, the incidence of post-PBMV restenosis ranged from 5 to 20%. Age, valve leaflet feature, NYHA stage, atrial fibrillation and transvalvular gradients, mitral valve orifice area, and mitral regurgitation are independent predictors of restenosis and long-term outcomes.

12.7.6 Other Complications

Postoperative arrhythmia occurs in 0.5–3.7% of PBMV, and residual shunt at the puncture site of atrial septum also occurs with a low incidence. 60% of patients with small shunt can disappear by themself [7, 8].

12.8 Technique Advantages

Echocardiography has a clear advantage over radiation guidance in assessing cardiac structure and hemodynamic. First, it is easier to locate the optimal puncture site under echocardiography guidance. The distance between puncture site and the MV can be adjusted according to atrial size, which facilitates balloon passing through the MV. Secondly, the relative position of the balloon and the heart structure is more visually visible under echocardiography, which makes it easier to adjust the direction of the balloon catheter during procedure, making it easier to pass through the narrow valve orifice. In contrast, the relative positional relationship between the catheter-guided tip and the mitral valve orifice is difficult to accurately judge under solely X-ray guidance. Again, echocardiography guidance can clearly show the entire process of balloon dilatation and determine if the position of the balloon is correct in real time. Under the X-ray, the valve cannot be clearly seen; during the expansion process, the balloon can easily drop into the left ventricle or the left atrium, and the effective expansion of the narrow valve cannot be achieved. Finally, post-expansion echocardiography can assess the dilatation effect, valvular regurgitation, and whether there is a combination of pericardial effusion and chordae damage.

12.9 Cases

Case 1 (Video 12.1) A 40-year-old female with 28 weeks pregnant. Her height was 160 cm.

Chief complaint: Palpitations, chest tightness, short of breath for 2 months, aggravation of 1 week.

Medical history: The patient was found to have moderate mitral stenosis with pulmonary hypertension, sinus rhythm, and dyspnea at 20 weeks of gestation.

Physical and laboratory examination: Blood pressure was 100/70 mmHg, heart rate was 90 beats/min, rales could be heard at both sides of chest, blood oxygen saturation was 92%. Echocardiography revealed a mitral valve orifice area (MVOA) was 0.7 cm^2; mean transvalvular pressure gradient (MVG) was 20 mmHg. The mitral valve mobility was good, with no calcification, a mild mitral regurgitation. No evidence of significant left atrial thrombus was found by TTE. The diagnosis was pregnancy with mitral stenosis; it was indication of mitral valvuloplasty under echocardiography, which could avoid the radiation of X-ray.

Methods: The patient was placed in a supine position, general anesthesia, and spontaneous breathing. Before procedure echocardiography was performed again to measure the mitral transvalvular pressure gradient and the valve orifice area. Punctured the right femoral vein, placed the 14F femoral vascular sheath, and advanced the 6F MPA2 catheter and guide wire through the vascular sheath. The Mullins sheath and the Brockenbrough needle were manipulated under echocardiography guidance to have their tips enter the atrial septal fossa ovals. After puncture, a small amount of saline was injected via the catheter to observe whether there was a cloud-like water bubble in the left atrium, and it was further verified whether the puncture was successful and whether the brockenbrough needle had entered the left atrium, and the pressure curve was also recorded. After confirming successful puncture, the left atrial guide wire was placed and the Inoue balloon catheter (26 mm) was passed through the left atrial guide wire. The direction of the balloon catheter was adjusted under echocardiography guidance. The distal end of balloon was entered the left ventricle across the mitral valve. The position of the balloon was adjusted under echocardiography guidance so that the balloon was located at the center of mitral valve, the balloon catheter was fixed, and the balloon was inflated rapidly to expand the mitral valve. The mitral valve was expanded twice with a diameter of 25 and 26 mm balloon, respectively. After the expansion was satisfactory, the catheter, the guide wire, and the arterial sheath were withdrawn, and compression bandages were applied.

Outcome: The diameter of the left atrium was reduced from 48 to 40 mm; the mean pressure of the left atrium was reduced from 20 to 11 mmHg. The mitral transvalvular pressure gradient was reduced from 14 to 7 mmHg. The mean postoperative pulmonary artery pressure was reduced to 15 mmHg. The mitral valve area was increased from 0.7 to 2.2 cm^2. The diastolic rumbling murmur was reduced from severe to mild, and the symptoms such as chest tightness and short of breath were significantly alleviated. The procedure time was 32 min. The intraoperative blood loss was 30 mL, and the patient was discharged from the hospital as early as 2 days after surgery. At 3 months follow-up, all symptoms disappeared.

Case 2 (Video 12.2) A 40-year-old female, her weight was 48 kg.

Chief complaint: Chest tightness, palpitations for 5 years, aggravation of 1 year.

Physical and laboratory examination:

Blood pressure was 115/63 mmHg, pulse was 64 beats/min, blood oxygen saturation was 98%, diastolic rumbling murmur was heard at apical area. ECG: left atrial enlargement, abnormal P wave; chest X-ray: congestion of two lungs. The heart-thorax ratio was 0.56. The heart shadow was pear-shaped and enlarged; the left atrium was obviously large. The echocardiogram showed that the mitral valve orifice area was 0.7 cm^2; mean transvalvular pressure gradient was 19 mmHg. The mitral valve leaflets were mild calcified with a mild mitral regurgitation. There was no thrombus detected in the left atrium by TEE examination. She had indication of percutaneous mitral valvuloplasty under transesophageal echocardiographic guidance.

Methods: The patient was placed in supine position with general anesthesia and intubation. Punctured the right femoral vein, placed the 14F femoral vascular sheath, and passed the 6F MPA2 catheter and guide wire through the vascular sheath. The sheath and the needle were manipulated under TEE guidance to have their tips enter the atrial septal fossa. After the catheter cross atrial septum, a small amount of microbubbles saline was injected into the catheter to observe whether there was a cloud-like water bubble in the left atrium, and it was further determined whether the puncture was successful and whether the brockenbrough needle had entered the left atrium, and the pressure curve was also recorded. After confirming successful puncture, the left atrial guide wire was placed and an Inoue balloon catheter (26 mm) was placed along the left atrial guide wire. The direction of the balloon catheter was adjusted under TEE guidance and sent the distal end of balloon catheter to enter the left ventricle the mitral valve. The position of the balloon was adjusted under TEE guidance so that the balloon was located at the center of mitral valve annulus, and fixed balloon catheter, the balloon was rapidly inflated to expand the mitral valve. The mitral valve was dilated three times with a 26 mm balloon. After the expansion was satisfactory, the catheter, the guide wire, and the arterial sheath were withdrawn; compression bandage was applied.

Outcome: Left atrial diameter was decreased from 47 to 40 mm, mean left atrial pressure was decreased from 19 to 10 mmHg, and the mitral transvalvular pressure gradient was reduced from 15 to 8 mmHg. The mean pulmonary arterial pressure was 25 mmHg post-PBMV. Mitral valve orifice area was increased from 0.7 to 1.8 cm^2, mitral valve diastolic murmur decreased from severe to mild, and the symptoms significantly improved. Procedural time was 35 min, and intraoperative bleeding volume was 20 mL. The patient was discharged 2 days after the operation. There were no complications during 3-months follow-up.

References

1. Silversides CK, et al. Cardiac risk in pregnant women with rheumatic mitral stenosis. Am J Cardiol. 2003;91(11):1382–5.
2. Chmielak Z, et al. Repeat percutaneous mitral balloon valvuloplasty for patients with mitral valve restenosis. Catheter Cardiovasc Interv. 2010;76(7):986–92.
3. Gupta A, et al. Balloon mitral valvotomy in pregnancy: maternal and fetal outcomes. J Am Coll Surg. 1998;187(4):409–15.
4. Elkayam U, Bitar F. Valvular heart disease and pregnancy part I: native valves. J Am Coll Cardiol. 2005;46(2):223–30.
5. Pan XB, Pang KJ, Hu SS, et al. Safety and efficacy of percutaneous transcatheter closure of atrial septal defect under transesophageal echocardiography guidance in children. Chin J Cardiol. 2013;41(9):744–6.
6. Wang H, YL L, Xiong JR, et al. Role of Doppler echocardiography in guidance of percutaneous balloon mitral valvuloplasty. Chin J Ultrason Imaging. 2004;10(11):648–50.
7. Baysson H, et al. Risk of cancer associated with cardiac catheterization procedures during childhood: a cohort study in France. BMC Public Health. 2013;13:266.
8. Meinel FG, et al. Radiation risks from cardiovascular imaging tests. Circulation. 2014;130(5):442–5.

Thromboembolism in atrial fibrillation typically caused by thrombi originating in the LAA, Although recent advances have been made in the field of systemic anticoagulation with the novel oral anticoagulants, these medications come with a significant risk for bleeding and are contraindicated in many patients. This has led to the development of LAA occlusion to reduce stroke risk in patients who have a contraindication to long-term oral anticoagulation therapy [1, 2].

13.1 Anatomy

The LAA is a finger-like extension originating from the main body of the left atrium which consists of three essential regions including ostium, neck, and body. The ostium region connects the LAA to the left atrium (LA). There is a large variability in the size and shape of the LAA, which affects clinical treatment. In most hearts the LAA is located above the left ventricle, anterior to the left pulmonary artery and ascending aorta, between the left superior pulmonary vein and the mitral annulus.

The most common LAA morphology is narrow and long tubular, with variable shapes. The volume of LAA ranges from 0.77 to 19.20 mL, and length ranges from 16 to 51 mm. The minimum diameter of LAA ostium ranges from 5 to 27 mm and maximum diameter ranges from 10 to 40 mm. Seventy percent of the LAA body is curved or spiral. The edge of the LAA is jagged and the 80% of the LAA body is multilobe. There are abundant pectinate muscles and trabeculae inside the LAA. Ninety-seven percent of pectinate muscles are larger than 1 mm in diameter. The LAA receives blood supply from the circumflex artery and right coronary artery and is governed by the sympathetic and vagal nerves.

The shapes of LAA were classified into 4 morphological types: "chicken wing" (an obvious bend in the proximal part of the dominant lobe), "windsock" (one dominant lobe acts as the primary structure), "cactus" (dominant central lobe with secondary lobes extending from the central lobe in the superior and inferior directions), and the "cauliflower" (limited overall length with more complex internal characteristics). The incidence of stroke is the lowest among patients with "chicken wing" and the highest among ones with cauliflower morphology [3].

13.2 Pathophysiology

In sinus rhythm, normal contraction and adequate blood flow within the LAA lower the risk for formation of thrombi inside its cavity. However, under the condition of AF, LA inner diameter and LA contraction intensity will increase in order to pump sufficient blood into the left ventricle. With the enlargement of the LA, there is a decrease in LAA contracility and function, which tends to cause low-velocity blood flow and vortexes, resulting in blood deposition and thrombosis. If AF lasts more than 48 h, a thrombus could be formed mostly attached in LAA. Thrombosis could lead to arterial embolism, 90% of which is cerebral arterial embolism (ischemic stroke), 10% is peripheral arterial embolism or mesenteric artery embolism [4, 5].

Electronic Supplementary Material The online version of this chapter (https://doi.org/10.1007/978-981-15-2055-6_13) contains supplementary material, which is available to authorized users.

13.3 Indications and Contraindications

13.3.1 Indications

According to ANMCO/AIAC/SICI-GISE/SIC/SICCH Consensus Document [6], the procedure is indicated in patients with non-valvular AF with high-thromboembolic risk (CHA$_2$DS$_2$-VASc score ≥2) (Table 13.1) with long-term contraindication for OAT (e.g. history of intracranial bleeding, life-threatening bleeding, coagulation diseases). Moreover, LAA occlusion could also be considered in the following clinical situations: patients with non-valvular AF with high-thromboembolic risk and high-haemorrhagic risk (HAS-BLED ≥3) (Table 13.2); patients requiring triple antithrombotic therapy indefinitely; patients with tumours with increased risk of haemorrhage, underestimated by the HAS-BLED score; patients in whom OAT is ineffective in providing protection against cerebral ischaemic events probably correlated to thromboembolisms originating from the LAA; patients with kidney failure or undergoing dialysis, all NOACs are contraindicated with creatinine clearance <15 mL/min and that in these patients warfarin could increase tissue calcification and the degree of atherosclerosis; patients with major bleeding of the urogenital or gastrointestinal system, or any other districts, such as the ocular area; frail patients (the very old, dementia, neurodegenerative diseases, malnutrition, etc.); patients with difficulty in managing oral therapies (e.g. mental illnesses, vision impairment); patients who, after being suitably informed about the OAT/NOACs therapy, refuse it and demand a 'definitive' therapy.

13.3.2 Contraindications

LA diameter >65 mm, TEE examination found intracardiac thrombosis or left atrial appendage thrombosis, severe mitral valve disease, pericardial effusion >3 mm, estimated survival <1 year, low risk of stroke and hemorrhage, AF combined with other disease requiring oral warfarin or surgery treatment, LVEF <35% or NYHA class IV and preoperative imaging examination shows that the LAA is not suitable for interventional occlusion.

Table 13.1 Stroke risk: CHA$_2$DS$_2$-VASc score

CHA$_2$DS$_2$-VASc		
	Condition	Points
C	Congestive heart failure (or left ventricular systolic dysfunction)	1
H	Hypertension: blood pressure consistently above 140/90 mmHg (or treated hypertension on medication)	1
A$_2$	Age ≥75 years	2
D	Diabetes mellitus	1
S$_2$	Prior stroke or TIA or thromboembolism	2
V	Vascular disease (e.g., peripheral artery disease, myocardial infarction, aortic plaque)	1
A	Age 65–74 years	1
Sc	Sex category (i.e., female sex)	1

The CHA$_2$DS$_2$-VASc score is a refinement of CHADS$_2$ [6, 7, 8] score and extends the latter by including additional common stroke risk factors, that is, age 65–74, female gender, and vascular disease [8]. In the CHA$_2$DS$_2$-VASc score, age 75 and above also has extra weight, with two points. The maximum CHADS$_2$ score is 6, while the maximum CHA$_2$DS$_2$-VASc score is 9 (not 10, as might be expected from simply adding up the columns; the maximum score for age is two points)

Table 13.2 Bleeding risk: HAS-BLED score

HAS-BLED		
	Condition	Points
H	Hypertension (SBP >160 mmHg)	1
A	Abnormal renal and liver function (1 point each)	1 or 2
S	Stroke	2
B	Bleeding tendency/predisposition	1
L	Labile INRs (if on warfarin)	2
E	Elderly (age >56 years)	1
D	Drugs or alcohol (1 point each)	1 or 2

13.4 Preoperative Examination

1. Detailed clinical examination include: assessment of clinical symptoms of atrial fibrillation, assessment of other cardiovascular diseases and cardiac function, stroke, and bleeding risk stratification.

2. Routine laboratory and imaging examinations: Chest X-ray, electrocardiogram, echocardiography, routine blood test, liver and kidney function and blood electrolytes, coagulation time and infectious disease indicators. The purpose of the examination is to comprehensively evaluate the function of the patient's heart and other organs, and if necessary, increase related items such as myocardial enzymes, pulmonary function tests, and Holter monitor electrocardiogram according to the condition.

3. Preoperative transthoracic (TTE) and/or transesophageal echocardiography (TEE) examination should focus on the following items: confirming no thrombus in the left atrial appendage or left atrium; measuring the size and depth of the left atrial appendage; assessing the left atrial appendage morphology. If necessary, a CT scan is required to confirm the anatomy to determine whether it is suitable for percutaneous left atrial appendage occlusion.

4. Sign the surgical informed consent before operation to inform the possibility of open heart surgery in critical condition and possible complications.

5. Preoperative intravenous infusion treatment to avoid left atrial appendage collapse and affect the mesurement accuracy.

13.5 Pre-procedural Imaging Preparation

In this procedure, how to choose an occluder without fluoroscopy and contrast agents is the key to success. We propose the choice of the LAmbre™ and ACP™ occluder under TEE guidance. The LAA orifice is defined as the plane connecting the ridge of pulmonary vein to the inferior junction of the left atrium and the LAA level of the left circumflex artery. The size and depth of the LAA is measured by preoperative TEE views at 0°, 45°, 90°, and 135° angles. The midpoint of the LAA orifice is marked as point A. TEE is performed at a 45° view to measure the distance (D1) from the left lower pulmonary vein to the point A and the distance (D2) from the mitral annulus to the point A. D1 or D2 (whichever the shorter distance) should be multiplied by 2. This gives the maximum diameter of the cover disc of the device to be used. The LAA landing zone is defined as an area approximately 1.5 cm from the point A, where a potential LAA device could be safely located in the body region of the appendage. A line across point A and perpendicular to the LAA orifice was drawn and the diameter (D3) of the LAA is measured at a distance of 1.5 cm from point A along the line. The diameter of the landing umbrella of occluder should be 6–8 mm larger than D3. If the selected landing umbrella was too large, the occluder will be stretched and the cover disc will not fully cover the LAA orifice. The occluder size is selected based on the above measurement results [9] (Fig. 13.1).

13.5.1 Device Preparation

16F puncture needle, 9F lower extremity arterial sheath, 6F multipurpose catheter (Cordis, 100 cm, 0.038 in. [0.965 mm]), Loach guide wire (260 cm), 71 cm transeptal needle and 8F SL1 puncture sheath (Mullins sheath), delivery system, LAA occluder, and pressure monitoring device.

13.5.2 Procedure

Patients were placed in supine position, routine general anesthesia with tracheal intubation, TEE examination before operation, measurement of left atrial appendage opening size and depth, distance from mitral valve and left lower pulmonary vein, selection of occluder and its appropriate delivery system. The diameter of the occluder cover disc is chosen to be 3–8 mm larger than the diameter of the orifice of the left atrial appendage. The position that the top 1/3 of the landing umbrella of the occluder would be deployed out of the delivery sheath is marked at the delivery cable. The right femoral vein is punctured, the distance between the right third intercostal parasternal space and the puncture site is measured as the working length in order to control the depth that the catheter should be inserted. A 9F arterial sheath is introduced through which a SL1 atrial septum puncture sheath (St. Jude) and guide wire are advanced under TEE guidance into the right atrium through the inferior vena cava. Then the guide wire is withdrawn. A transeptal needle was inserted through the sheath, which is positioned at the posterior and inferior part of the atrial septum towards LAA under TEE guidance using the apical four-chamber and parasternal short-axis views. After transeptal puncture, heparin (80–100 U/Kg) is administrated. Then the guide wire is inserted into the left atrium, the SL1 sheath is withdrawn, and the depth that the SL1 sheath has been inserted is measured. The delivery system is inserted into the left atrium along the guide wire according to the distance. The guide wire and the inner core are withdrawn while maintaining the delivery sheath in the left atrium. The pigtail catheter is inserted through

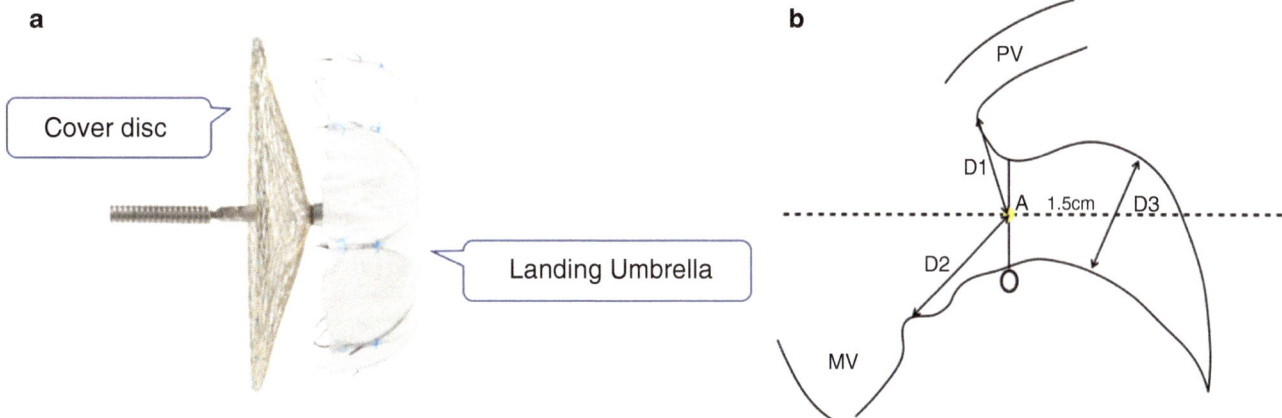

Fig. 13.1 (**a**) The structure of LAmbre™ left atrial appendage occluder. (**b**) Schematic diagram of the left atrial appendage measurement

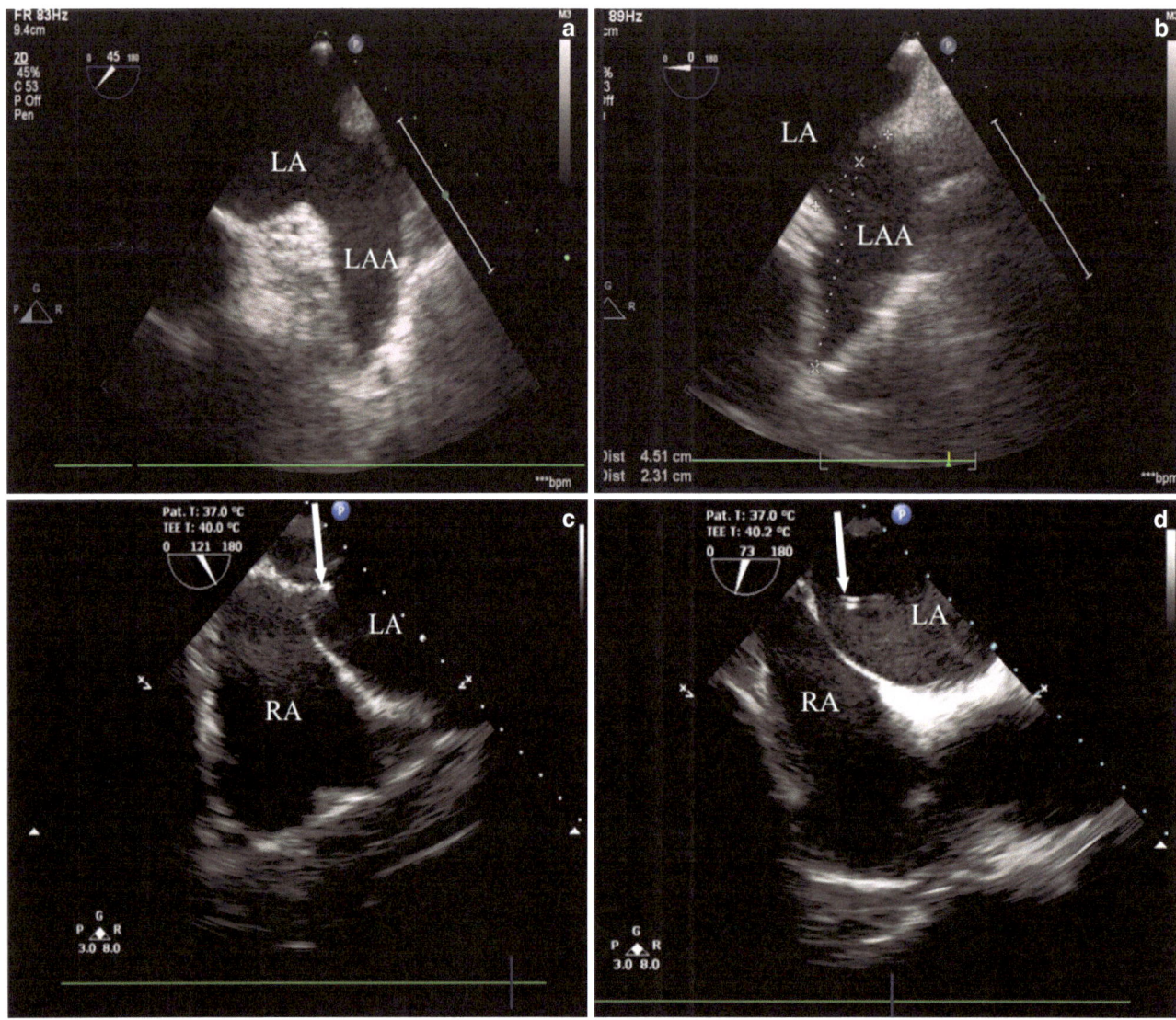

Fig. 13.2 Transesophageal echocardiography: (**a**) Shows left atrium and left atrial appendage. (**b**) Shows the measurements of the size and depth of the left atrial appendage. (**c**) Shows punctured interatrial sep- tum (↑), the image can be seen as a tent-like protrusion. (**d**) Shows the puncture sheath (↑) is in left atrium through atrial septum

the delivery system and steered into the left atrium append- age and the delivery system is inserted into the left atrium appendage along the pigtail catheter. The LAA occluder is inserted along the delivery sheath. Top 1/3 of the landing umbrella is deployed out of the delivery sheath according to the marker on the cable, adjust the position of the deliv- ery sheath and ensure that the top of landing umbrella reach the landing zone. The delivery cable is fixed, the delivery sheath is retrieved, and the occluder is deployed under TEE monitoring. A push-pull test is performed to verify its stability. TEE is used to detect residual leakage, mitral regurgitation, left inferior pulmonary vein blood flow and pericardial effusion and to confirm occluder mor- phology and position. The delivery cable is rotated coun- terclockwise to release the occluder. If the patient also has

an atrial septal defect suitable for percutaneous closure, an atrial septal defect occluder could also be implanted under echocardiographic guidance. After reconfirming the posi- tion and shape of the occluder by TEE, the delivery system was withdrawn. The puncture site is sutured and bandaged [10] (Figs. 13.2 and 13.3).

13.6   Postoperative Care

The puncture site should be compressed for 4 h after proce- dure. The patients should stay in bed for 12 h. The ECG, vital signs, heart rate, blood pressure, and oxygen saturation should be monitored for 24 h to find the changes of the patient's condition and to give therapy in time. Puncture site

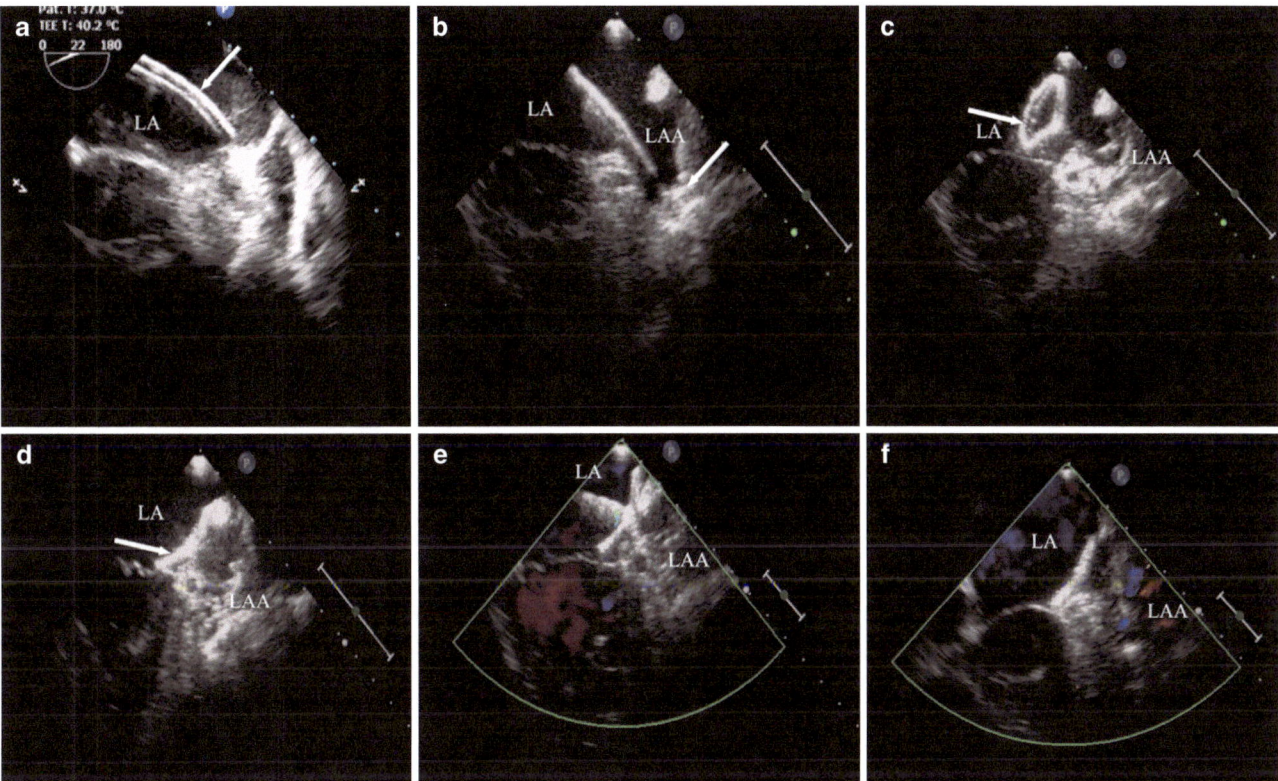

Fig. 13.3 Transesophageal echocardiography showed left atrial appendage sealing process: (**a**) The occluder delivery sheath (↑) is in the left atrium. (**b**) left atrial appendage occluder first umbrella disc (↑) is deployed. (**c**) left atrial appendage occluder second umbrella disc (↑) was partially deployed. (**d**) Left atrial appendage occluder (↑) was deployed. (**e**) Doppler examination indicates no residual leakage. (**f**) Occluder was completely released

should be examined to find hematoma and the pulsation of the dorsal artery of the foot should be examined carefully, to prevent the lower extremity ischemia caused by the compression on the puncture site. Low-molecular heparin is administered subcutaneously 24 h post-procedure. Oral aspirin 100 mg/d and Plavix 75 mg/d were given for 6 months from the second day after procedure. Antibiotics are given intravenously once half an hour pre-procedure and 6 h post-procedure. The echocardiography, electrocardiogram, and chest X-ray should be performed within 24 h after procedure. All patients will be followed up at 1, 3, 6, and 12 months after procedure.

13.7   Postoperative Complications and Treatment

13.7.1   Pericardial Effusion

Because the left atrial appendage belongs to the residual attachment of the left atrium, its thickness is uneven, and the thinnest area of the LAA wall is extremely easy to break. In the operation of the occlusion, guide wire catheter operation, atrial septal puncture, etc. may cause LAA dam-

age, resulting in pericardial effusion. A large amount of pericardial effusion may cause pericardial tamponade, and immediate pericardial puncture drainage is needed. If pericardial effusion occurs, the mangement depending upon the size of effusion and clinical presentation, effusion without evidence of tamponade requires non-urgent treatment while effusions presenting as pericardial tamponade need urgent approach. In patients with small amount of pericardial effusion, the vital signs should be observed. If the patient's vital signs are stable, the LAA occlusion could continue to be performed.

13.7.2   Occluder Displacement

The incidence rate of occluder displacement is about 4%. The occluder displacement can cause serious complications and even sudden death. It is very important to choose the appropriate size of the occluder and the correct position of the occluder. After the occluder is released, it needs to be checked again. The stability of the occluder should be confirmed by push-pull test. Once the occluder is detached, it is necessary to perform a thoracotomy to remove it by surgeons.

13.7.3 Residual Shunt

Since the occluder device is circular and the left atrial appendage orifice is generally elliptical, there is theoretically the possibility of residual leakage. The severity of residual leakage can be assessed by color Doppler and divided into severe (multiple beams of shunts, or the width of shunt flow was >3 mm); medium (the width of shunt flow was 1–3 mm); mild (the width of shunt flow was <1 mm); no residual leakage (no shunt flow). The incidence of residual leaks was about 5%, and most of them are mild residual leaks, and their effects are negligible.

13.7.4 Other Complications

13.7.4.1 Esophageal Injury

Esophageal mucosal injury: Esophageal mucosal damage is mainly caused by mal-operation. In order to avoid iatrogenic injury, it is necessary to accurately adjust the position of the device before the operation, and check whether there is foreign matter on the probe, whether the lubricant is sufficient, whether there is bloodshot on the probe after inspection, and pay close attention to whether the operation is gentle.

13.7.4.2 Air Embolism

Air embolism may occur during procedures. Operation process should be manipulated carefully to reduce the risk of air embolism. The delivery sheath should be filled with heparinized saline, an appropriate size occluder should be used, and the end of the delivery sheath should be kept under water when inserting the occluder.

13.7.4.3 Residual Atrial Septal Shunt

Residual shunt may occur at the position of atrial septal puncture. Its incidence is low and 60% of patients can self-heal.

13.8 Technical Advantages

Existing LAA occlusion devices (such as LAmbre, ACP, and WATCHMAN) are already available to be implanted under echocardiography guidance. Echocardiography has a clear advantage over radiation in assessing cardiac structure and hemodynamic. Under the guidance of transesophageal echocardiography, the heart structure can be clearly displayed, and the diameter of the left atrial appendage in cardiac cycle and normal filling state can be measured. The puncture point can be accurately located during the interatrial septum puncture, and the puncture point located in the lower part of the interatrial septum can facilitate advancing the sheath into LAA,

because the sheath enters the left atrial appendage at a small angle. Echocardiographic positioning can also avoid damage to the aorta and other important structures. During the release of the occluder, the echocardiography image can accurately display the position and shape of the occluder in real time, which will be beneficial to avoid the occluder being placed too deep or too shallow and to prevent obstructing the mitral valve or pulmonary veins. Of course, due to the echocardiographic section-type exploration method, the multiplane scan needs to be repeated for the judgment of the position of the tip end of the catheter guide wire. The cooperation between the sonographer and the operator is very important. Transthoracic ultrasound has limited detection of the left atrial appendage. Even in the traditional radiation-guided mode, transesophageal echocardiography should be used. However, it does not mean that transthoracic echocardiography cannot guide percutaneous left atrial appendage. For patients with clear acoustic windows, the procedure can be guided with transthoracic echocardiography.

13.9 Cases

Case 1 The patient is a 73-year-old female (Video 13.1).

Chief complaint: 2 years of recurrent palpitations and chest tightness.

History: The patient has had a stroke and occasionally took warfarin. The patient has a history of hypertension and kidney dysfunction.

Preoperative examination: HR, 85/min; BP, 165/100 mmHg. ECG diagnosis was atrial fibrillation. CHA_2DS_2-VASc score was 5 points. TEE: No thrombus was found in the left atrium and LAA, the shape of LAA structure is suitable for left atrial appendage occlusion.

Admission diagnosis: (1) persistent atrial fibrillation; (2) primary hypertension; (3) chronic renal failure; (4) old cerebral infarction; (5) Multiple atherosclerosis with plaque formation; (6) chronic gastritis.

Due to kidney dysfunction of the patient, the echocardiography-guided percutaneous interventions for left atrial appendage occlusion was referred.

Procedure: The patient was placed in supine position, general anesthesia, and tracheal intubation. The transesophageal echocardiography was performed before procedure, and the left atrial appendage orifice and depth were measured. The LAA orifice was 23 mm × 30 mm. The right femoral vein was punctured, the 9Fr sheath was placed, and the MPA2 catheter and guide wire were delivered through the arterial sheath. The MPA2 catheter tip was localized to the fossa ovalis under TEE guidance; the guide wire then was kept inside, and the catheter removed. A Mullins catheter (SL1) was inserted along the guide wire. A transeptal puncture needle was used for transeptal puncture. Heparin was injected. The guide wire was positioned in the left atrium, and the delivery sheath was inserted along the guide wire into the left atrium. The LAA occluder was inserted along the delivery sheath. Top 1/3 of the landing umbrella was deployed out of the delivery sheath, advance the delivery sheath, and ensure that the top of landing umbrella reach the landing zone. The occluder was implanted under TEE monitoring. A push-pull test was performed. There were no complications.

Outcome: No residual shunt. Procedural time was 1 h, and intraoperative bleeding volume was 20 mL. The patient was discharged 2 days after procedure. The patient was followed up at 45 days after procedure, the TEE was performed and showed that the occluder was in good position without residual shunt. The patient was given oral aspirin and Plavix for 6 months after procedure. The patient had no complications.

Case 2 The patient is 71-year-old male (Video 13.2).

Chief complaint: After the activity, feel chest tightness, and shortness of breath for 5 years.

History: Cerebral infarction occurred 2 years ago. After that, the left extremity was weak and the speech was unclear.

Physical examination: HR, 90/min; BP, 155/90 mmHg. EKG: Atrial fibrillation. CHA_2DS_2-VASc score was 4 points. TEE: ASD (central type) with good edges and left-to-right shunt. No thrombus was found in the left atrium and LAA, and the type of LAA structure was suitable for left atrial appendage occlusion.

Procedure: The patient was placed in supine position, general anesthesia, and tracheal intubation. The transesophageal echocardiography was performed before surgery, and the left atrial appendage orifice and depth were measured. The ASD was 26 mm. The LAA orifice was 21 mm × 29 mm. The right femoral vein was punctured and a 9F sheath was placed and a multifunctional catheter and guide wire were delivered. Transeptal puncture under echocardiographic guidance was performed. After the puncture atrial septum, the guide wire was placed into the left atrium, and the delivery system would be advanced into the left atrium along the guide wire, and then the guide wire and the inner core are withdrawn, and the delivery sheath is left in the left atrium. The occluder (LAmbre™) was inserted into the left atrial appendage through the delivery sheath. Then observe if residual leakage or mitral valve regurgitation occurs, measure the blood flow in the left lower pulmonary vein and check for signs of pericardial effusion by transesophageal echocardiography. After confirmation that the occluder was in good shape and position, rotate the push rod counter clockwise and release the occluder, the delivery sheath was withdrawn and exchanged with a 14F long sheath, and a

36 mm ASD occluder was placed in the atrial septum. After the good results are confirmed, withdraw the delivery system. Bandage the site of puncture and compressed to stop bleeding.

Outcome: Color Doppler showed no significant residual shunt from LAA occluder, or ASD occluder. The procedure time was 65 min, and the intraoperative blood loss was 30 mL. The patient was discharged 2 days after the procedure. The patient was followed up on 45 days after procedure, TEE examination confirmed the occluder was in good position, no significant residual shunt, no thrombus on the surface of the device, and double anticoagulation (oral aspirin + clopidogrel) for 6 months after procedure.

Case 3 The patient is 65-year-old male.

Chief complaint: 1 year of recurrent palpitations.

History: Cerebral infarction occurred 1 year ago. The patient has a history of gastric bleeding for 1 year. The patient has a history of kidney dysfunction.

Physical examination: HR, 98/min; BP, 140/90 mmHg. EKG: Atrial fibrillation. CHA_2DS_2-VASc score was three points. TEE: No thrombus was found in the left atrium and LAA, the shape of LAA structure is suitable for left atrial appendage occlusion.

Procedure: The patient was placed in supine position, general anesthesia, and tracheal intubation. The transesophageal echocardiography was performed before surgery, and the left atrial appendage orifice and depth were measured. The LAA orifice was 20 mm. The right femoral vein was punctured, the 9Fr sheath was placed, and the MPA2 catheter and guide wire were delivered through the arterial sheath. The tip of the MPA2 catheter was localized to the fossa ovalis under TEE guidance; the guide wire then was kept inside, and the catheter was removed. A Mullins catheter (SL1) was inserted along the guide wire. A transeptal puncture needle was used for transeptal puncture. After the puncture, heparin was injected. The guide wire was positioned in the left atrium, and the delivery sheath was inserted along the guide wire into the left atrium. The LAA occluder (WATCHMAN) was inserted along the delivery sheath. The occluder was deployed out of the delivery sheath, advance the delivery sheath and ensure that the occluder reach the landing zone. The occluder was implanted under TEE monitoring. A push-pull test was performed. There were no complications.

Outcome: No residual shunt. Procedural time was 1 h, and intraoperative bleeding volume was 25 mL. The patient was discharged 2 days after procedure. The patient was followed up at 45 days after procedure, the TEE was performed and showed that the occluder was in good position without residual shunt. The patient was given oral aspirin and Plavix for 6 months after procedure. The patient had no complications.

References

1. Blackshear JL, Odell JA. Appendage obliteration to reduce stroke in cardiac surgical patients with atrial fibrillation. Ann Thorac Surg. 1996;61(2):755–9.
2. Ostermayer S, et al. Percutaneous closure of the left atrial appendage. J Interv Cardiol. 2003;16(6):553–6.
3. Spivey CA, et al. Stroke associated with discontinuation of warfarin therapy for atrial fibrillation. Curr Med Res Opin. 2015;31(11):2021–9.
4. Furberg CD, et al. Prevalence of atrial fibrillation in elderly subjects (the cardiovascular health study). Am J Cardiol. 1994;74(3):236–41.
5. Wann LS, et al. ACCF/AHA/HRS focused update on the management of patients with atrial fibrillation (update on dabigatran): a report of the American College of Cardiology Foundation/American Heart Association Task Force on practice guidelines. J Am Coll Cardiol. 2011;57(11):1330–7.
6. Casu G, Gulizia MM, Molon G, et al. ANMCO/AIAC/SICI-GISE/SIC/SICCH Consensus Document: percutaneous occlusion of the left atrial appendage in non-valvular atrial fibrillation patients: indications, patient selection, staff skills, organisation, and training[J]. European Heart Journal Supplements, 2017;19(suppl_D):D333–D353.
7. Sandhu RK, Bakal JA, Ezekowitz JA, McAlister FA. Risk stratification schemes, anticoagulation use and outcomes: the risk-treatment paradox in patients with newly diagnosed non-valvular atrial fibrillation. Heart. 2011;97(24):2046–50.
8. UCSF Cardiology|Atrial Fibrillation Medical Management. cardiology.ucsf.edu. Accessed 12 Feb 2017.
9. Holmes DR, et al. Percutaneous closure of the left atrial appendage versus warfarin therapy for prevention of stroke in patients with atrial fibrillation: a randomised non-inferiority trial. Lancet. 2009;374(9689):534–42.
10. Reddy VY, et al. Percutaneous left atrial appendage closure for stroke prophylaxis in patients with atrial fibrillation: 2.3-year follow-up of the PROTECT AF (Watchman left atrial appendage system for embolic protection in patients with atrial fibrillation) trial. Circulation. 2013;127(6):720–9.

Coarctation of the aorta (CoA) is a relatively rare congenital vascular malformation, which is mainly treated with surgical operation, balloon dilatation, and stent implantation. The preferred treatment is surgery. Balloon dilatation and stent implantation are mostly used for the treatment of postoperative restenosis. Due to the undesirable long-term effects of percutaneous balloon dilatation in the treatment of CoA, stent implantation is now favored in more clinical practice. Traditional balloon dilatation and stent implantation were performed under fluoroscopy guidance, while nowadays, the tries of using echocardiography as substitution could protect both patients and healthcare professionals from radiation and contrast agents, which would play an increasingly important role and have a promising future [1]. This chapter introduces how to perform PAN procedure for CoA.

14.1 Anatomical Features

Most stenosis of CoA locates at the aortic isthmus. According to the anatomical relationship of the stenosis and the arterial ligament or arterial duct, the lesion was divided into pre ductal-type and post ductal-type.

- Pre ductal-type: This type is relatively rare. The lesions locate at the proximal end of the arterial ligament or arterial duct, which would be relatively long, and probably complicated with patent ductus arteriosus (PDA). Severe cases would die of cardiac failure in infancy and early childhood if without appropriate treatment, so this type was also named infantile-type.
- Post ductal-type: This type is more common. The lesions locate at the aortic isthmus distal of the left subclavian artery origin. They tend to be short and localized, and

most cases have a closed arterial duct. Most patients with this type would survive till their adulthood. The proximal and distal aorta would distend to different extents and generate abundant collateral vessels. In this chapter, we mainly introduce the post ductal-type of CoA.

14.2 Pathophysiology

CoA results in increased blood flow resistance and thus leads to a pre-stenotic hypertension as while as the existence of post-stenotic hypotension, so for those patients, their blood pressure of upper extremity would be significantly higher than lower extremity. On the other hand, abundant collateral circulation is formed among the peri-stenotic area since fetus period to increase the blood supply for the distal arteries. The presence of hypertension and collateral circulation could probably lead to congestive heart failure, infective endocarditis, aortic rupture, cerebrovascular disease, etc.

14.3 Indications (Fig. 14.1)

- Postoperative restenosis, the type of constriction segment is suitable for interventional therapy, and systolic blood pressure gradient across the stenosis measured by catheter >20 mmHg.
- Postoperative restenosis, the type of constriction segment is suitable for interventional therapy, systolic blood pressure gradient across the stenosis measured by catheter <20 mmHg, but with one of the following conditions: obvious collateral angiogenesis, single ventricular circulation, or decreased left ventricular systolic function.
- CoA Patients with surgical contraindications without history of surgery.
- Discrete membranous CoA, without history of surgery, and systolic blood pressure gradient across the stenosis measured by catheter >20 mmHg [2].

Electronic Supplementary Material The online version of this chapter (https://doi.org/10.1007/978-981-15-2055-6_14) contains supplementary material, which is available to authorized users.

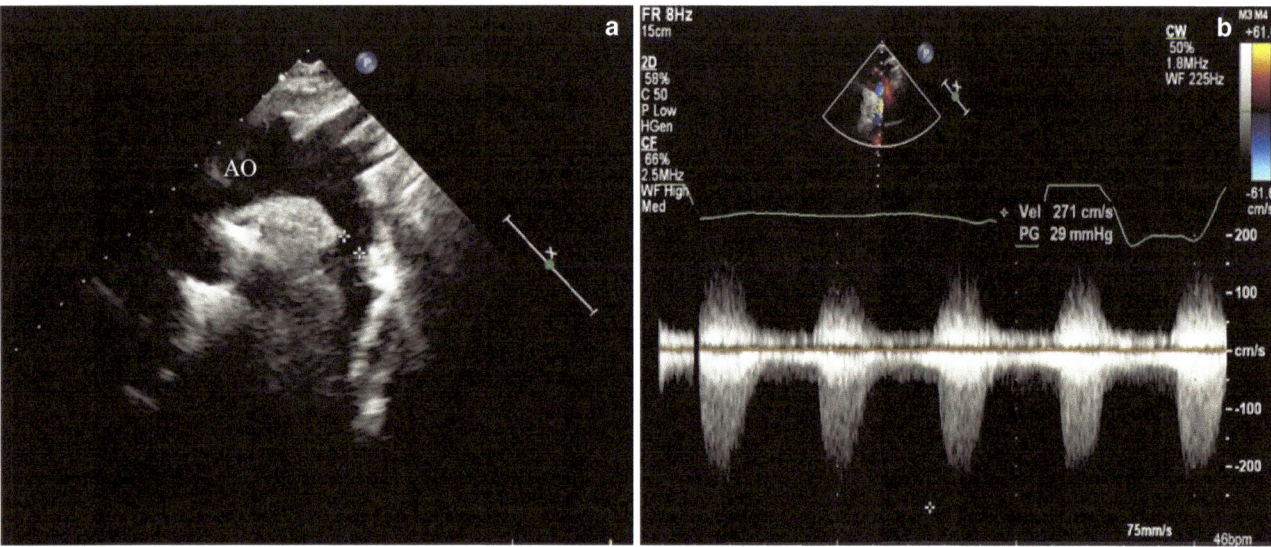

Fig. 14.1 Transthoracic echocardiography: (**a**) the suprasternal long-axis view of aortic arch shows the stenosis was at proximal thoracic aorta; (**b**) The blood pressure gradient across the stenosis is about 29 mmHg measured by continuous wave Doppler echocardiogram (anesthetic state)

14.4   Procedure

14.4.1   Pre-procedural Preparation

- Conventional laboratory and imaging examination items: X-ray film, multi-slice spiral CT (MDCT), electrocardiogram, echocardiography, blood routine, liver and kidney function and blood electrolytes, coagulation function and infectious disease indicators, and so on.
- Physical examination: Especially pay attention to measure upper and lower extremity blood pressure. The purpose of the examination is to comprehensively evaluate the function of the patient's heart and other organs, and if necessary, increase related items such as myocardial enzymes, pulmonary function tests, and Holter monitor according to the condition. Cardiac MDCT examination focuses on the initial assessment of the stenosis, the total length and inner diameter of the stenosis, the distance from the stenosis to the subclavian artery, the diameter of the ascending aorta, and the diameter of the aorta at the level of the diaphragm to guide the choice of the stent and balloon. The surgical informed consent form was signed before operation to inform the relevant risks and possible complications.
- Selection of interventional instruments: Interventional instruments often use CP stent grafts and BIB balloons. The length of the stent is selected according to the length of the narrow segment. Usually the length of the stent needs to exceed the length of the narrow segment. Currently, the length of the existing CP stent is 2.2, 2.8, 3.4, 3.9, and 4.5 cm; the diameter of the BIB balloon is the same as the diameter of the aorta at the diaphragm. Procedure can be

performed under transthoracic and/or 3D intravascular echocardiogram. To overcome the problem of accurate positioning of the catheter guide wire under echocardiography, it is recommended to use an interventional guide wire designed for echocardiography guidance (Fig. 4.1). The guide wire has a spindle-shaped head for accurate positioning under ultrasound.

14.4.2   Procedure

- Device preparation: 16G trocar, 6F/11F lower extremity arterial sheath, 6F multipurpose catheter (MPA2), Novel echocardiographic guide wire (Panna™ Wire), BIB balloon and CP stent, pressure monitor device, etc.
- Anesthesia: The patient was placed in the supine position with general anesthesia, and the radial artery and the dorsal artery of the foot were punctured for blood pressure monitoring.
- Femoral artery and vein puncture: After satisfactory anesthesia, use the 16G trocar to puncture the right femoral artery and the left femoral vein (prepared for intravascular echocardiography). The 6F lower extremity arterial sheath was placed through the right femoral artery, and the 11F lower extremity arterial sheath was placed through the left femoral vein (if intracardiac echocardiography device is available).
- A 3D intravascular echocardiography probe was placed through the left 11F lower extremity arterial sheath, and a 6F MPA2 catheter and guide wire were delivered through the 6F arterial sheath. The catheter and guide wire were placed into the aortic arch under transthoracic echocar-

diography guidance, and intracardiac echocardiography was performed. The probe was placed into the inferior vena cava into the right atrium. The stenosis was located by transthoracic and intracardiac echocardiography synergistically, and the diameter and length of the stenosis were measured again. Intracardiac echocardiography is not mandatory.

- Under echocardiography guidance, the super-stiff guide wire was passed through the aortic constriction section, into the ascending aorta. MPA2 catheter was then advanced into ascending aorta, the super-stiff guide wire was withdrawn, and the echocardiography-guided special guide wire (Panna™ wire) is inserted along the multipurpose catheter (MPA2). The tip of the Panna™ wire could expand into a diamond shape and the echocardiography can accurately confirm its location. Hold the guide wire, exit the MPA2 catheter and the 6F arterial sheath, place the COOK 12F delivery sheath into femoral artery, choose the appropriate stent and balloon according to the preoperative MDCT and intraoperative echocardiographyic measurements, and mount the stent on the balloon along the guide wire. Then the stent and the balloon are placed in the delivery sheath, the tip of the balloon is closely attached to the swollen portion of guide wire, the starting position of the stent is accurately positioned through the tip of the Panna™ guide wire under echocardiography guidance, and the BIB balloon is pressurized first after the position is satisfactory. The inner balloon expands the stent partially, and use the echocardiography scans again to confirm the position of the stent. If the stent is in poor position, the balloon catheter can be adjusted. During the period, it was necessary to ensure that the inner balloon was always in an inflated state, and after the positioning is accurate, then rapidly inflating the outer balloon to completely expand the stent. After the balloon was fully inflated. The balloon and the guide wire were withdrawn, and the multipurpose catheter (MPA2) was placed to measure the pressure. If the pressure measurement was unsatisfactory, the balloon could be expanded again. After the end of the operation, the femoral artery was pressure-wrapped and the femoral artery puncture site was sutured with a vascular suturing device (refer to Fig. 14.2).

It should be noted that the treatment can be completed with a normal super-stiff guide wire, but in the absence of Panna™ wire, the distance from the proximal of the stenosis to the subclavian artery should be accurately measured. Carefully identify the tip of the balloon catheter and the proximal end of the stent under echocardiography. Reconfirm the stent position by measure the corresponding distance [3, 4].

14.4.3 Post-procedural Care

The patient should rest in bed for 12 h, and the blood pressure, electrocardiogram, heart rate, and blood oxygen saturation should be monitored in order to detect any complication and give correct therapy in time. And pay attention to observe whether there is hematoma in the puncture site and the pulsation of the dorsal artery to prevent the lower extremity ischemia caused by the compression. All patients should take echocardiography, electrocardiogram, and chest X-ray within 24 h after procedure. The patients should be followed up with echocardiography at 1, 3, 6, and 12 months after procedure.

14.4.4 Efficacy Evaluation

The shape and location of the stents could be observed by transthoracic and intracardiac echocardiography after implantation. The gradient could be measured with catheter during or after procedure.

14.5 Complications

1. Thrombosis in femoral artery:
   Systemic heparinization therapy or urokinase can be given for thrombolysis. If drug therapy fails, catheterization or surgery should be performed for thrombus extraction.
2. Aortic dissection and aneurysm formation:
   The incidence of aortic dissection and aneurysm formation is reported differently. There were fewer aneurysms immediately after procedure and higher incidence of aneurysms during follow up.
3. Aortic rupture or perforation: Relatively rare. Once the guide wire or catheter has been found to have deviated from the aortic and archways, the catheter should be maintained in place and withdrawing blood from the catheter. If it is determined that the aorta has been perforated, the breathing and circulation state should be monitored closely, and the emergency thoracotomy should be performed.

14.6 Cases

Case 1 Patient is a 17-year-old girl, height was 164 cm, weight was 56 kg (Video 14.1).

Chief Complaint: Repeated dizziness for 1 year, syncope 1 time.

Physical examination and evaluation: Heart rate was 88 beats/min, oxygen saturation was 99%, blood pressure of left upper extremity was 140/79 mmHg, left lower extremity was

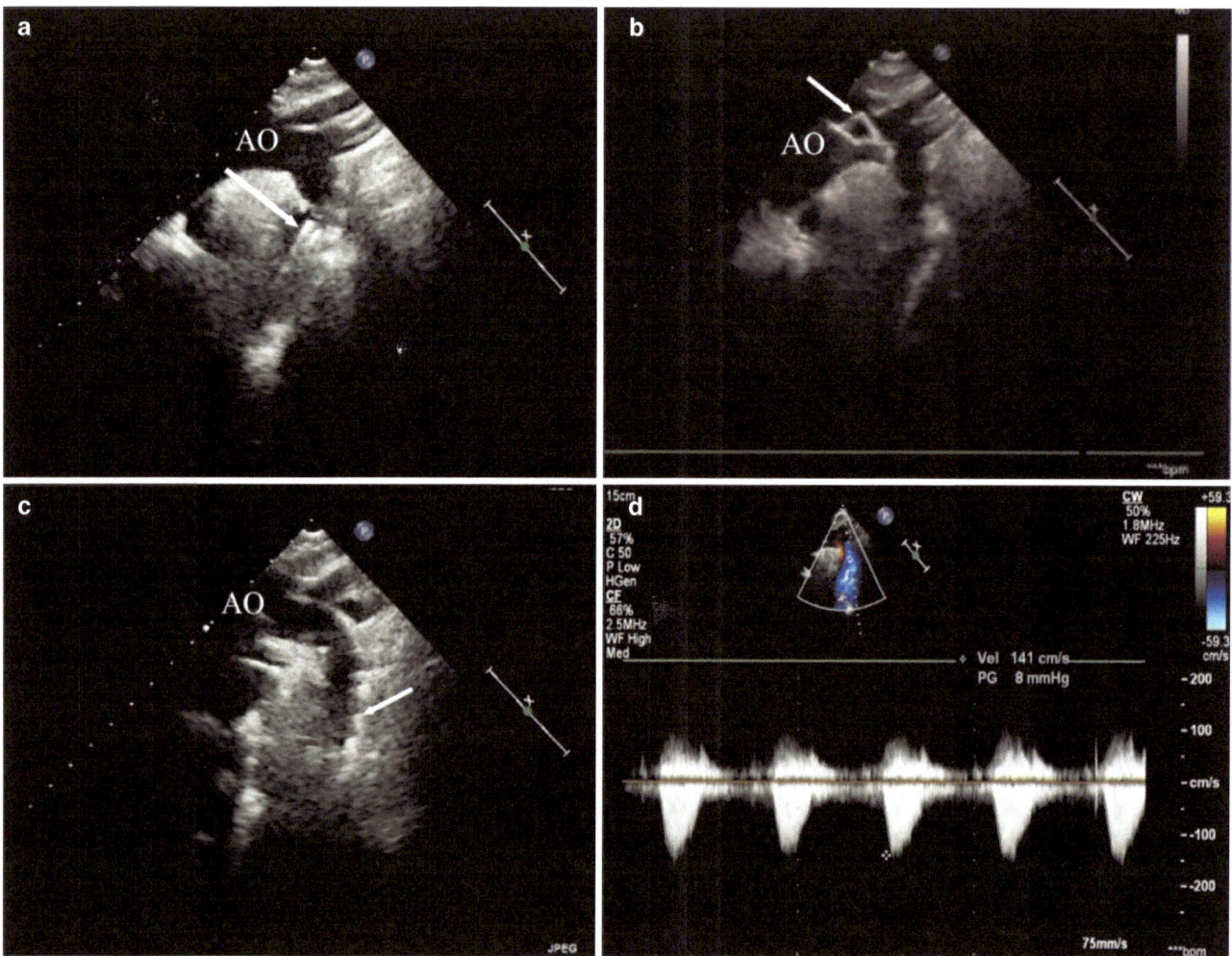

Fig. 14.2 Completely transthoracic echocardiography-guided CoA stent implantation. (**a**) The catheter (↑) reached the constriction area through the femoral artery. (**b**) Novel echocardiographic guide wire (Panna™ wire) entered the ascending aorta through the stenosis, and the echocardiography shows its spindle-shaped head (↑). (**c**) Stent (↑) was deployed. (**d**) The forward peak pressure gradient at proximal thoracic aorta was measured immediately after the stent implantation, which is about 8 mmHg

98/67 mmHg, right upper extremity was 132/76 mmHg, right lower extremity was 97/64 mmHg. Echocardiogram showed that the inner diameter of the ascending aorta was 23 mm, the inner diameter of the arch was about 22 mm, the isthmus of the aortic arch was distorted, and the inner diameter of the narrowest part was 10 mm. The descending distal aorta was slightly dilated. The aortic isthmus stenosis has a flow rate of about 4.1 m/s and a peak pressure gradient was about 64 mmHg. CT findings: localized aortic arch isthmus folds, stenosis, 10 mm at the narrowest point, with a diameter of 25 mm in distal aortic stenosis, a diameter of 20 mm in the middle of the ascending aorta, and a diameter of 21 mm in the lower part of the descending aorta.

Diagnosis: Congenital heart disease, aortic arch constriction. Percutaneous guided aortic arch constriction stent implantation under ultrasound guidance will be performed for therapy.

Procedure: The patient was placed in a supine position, general anesthesia, and tracheal intubation. Puncture of the radial artery and dorsal artery was performed for monitoring blood pressure. The upper extremity arterial pressure was 151/88 mmHg, and the left lower extremity arterial pressure was 99/62 mmHg. 16G trocar was inserted into the right femoral artery, placed into the 6F lower extremity arterial sheath, and the 6F multipurpose catheter (MPA2) and super-stiff guide wire were delivered through the arterial sheath. The super-stiff guide wire was passed through the aortic constriction under transthoracic echocardiography guidance. Into the ascending aorta, the multipurpose catheter (MPA2) is delivered along the guide wire, the super-stiff guide wire is withdrawn, and the special guide wire for echocardiography guidance is sent along the multipurpose catheter (MPA2). The head is expanded into a diamond shape, and the echocardiography can accurately locate its position. The guide wire was fixed, the multipurpose catheter (MPA2) and the 6F arterial sheath were withdrawn, and the COOK 14F delivery sheath was placed. Select 20 mm BIB balloon and 3.9 cm CP stent graft, mount the stent on the balloon, place the stent and balloon into the delivery sheath along the guide wire, and the balloon tip is close to the bulk of the guide wire tip and is guided by echocardiography. The initial position of the stent was accurately positioned through the enlarged guide wire tip end. After adjusting the stent to a satisfactory position, the balloon inner capsule and the outer balloon expansion stent were sequentially expanded, and the pressure was measured again. The upper extremity arterial pressure was 104/56 mmHg, and the lower extremity arterial pressure was 92/49 mmHg. Transthoracic echocardiography indicates that the position and shape of the stent are good. The catheter, guide wire, and arterial sheath were removed and the femoral artery puncture site was sutured with a vascular suturing device.

Therapeutic effect: The patient's dizziness symptoms were significantly improved. Echocardiography showed a laminar blood flow in the descending aortic stent with a velocity of blood flow of 2.3 m/s. The operation time was 25 min; the intraoperative blood loss was 40 mL, and the patient was discharged 2 days after procedure. The patient was followed up at 1 month after procedure and she was symptom free.

Case 2 Patient was a 26-year-old female, height was 152 cm, weight was 47 kg (Video 14.2).

Chief complaint: Recurrent amaurosis for 3 months and syncope once.

Physical and laboratory examination: Heart rate was 80 beats/min, oxygen saturation was 99%, blood pressure of left upper extremity was 157/82 mmHg, left lower extremity was 96/64 mmHg, right upper extremity was 148/78 mmHg, and right lower extremity was 98/66 mmHg. Echocardiography examination showed that the inner diameter of the aortic arch was 9 mm at the narrowest point, and the descending aorta was slightly dilated. The velocity of blood flow across the aortic stenosis was about 4.5 m/s, the peak pressure gradient was about 81 mmHg, and the patent ductus arteriosus was about 3 mm.

CT scan: The thinnest part of the aortic arch is located between the left common carotid artery and the left subclavian artery. The inner diameter is about 11.2 mm. The diameter of the left subclavian artery is about 15 mm. The aortic isthmus is severely narrow, with a minimum diameter of about 4 mm. A long patent duct artery with a diameter of about 3.5 mm was attached to the initial segment of the left pulmonary artery. The descending aorta was slightly dilated and nearly 15 mm in diameter; the main pulmonary artery was 24 mm, and the descending aorta was 12 mm.

Diagnosis: congenital heart disease, aortic arch constriction, patent ductus arteriosus. Percutaneous aortic arch constriction stent implantation under echocardiography guidance will be performed.

Procedure: The patient was placed in supine position with general anesthesia and tracheal intubation. The right radial and the dorsal pedis arteries were punctured for monitoring

blood pressure. The upper extremity blood pressure was 162/94 mmHg, and the lower extremity blood pressure was 98/65 mmHg. 16G trocar was inserted into the right femoral artery and placed into the 6F lower extremity arterial sheath, and the 6F MPA2 catheter and super-stiff guide wire were delivered through the arterial sheath. The super-stiff guide wire was passed through the aortic constriction into the ascending aorta under transthoracic echocardiography guidance, the MPA2 catheter is delivered along the guide wire, and then the super-stiff guide wire is withdrawn, and the special guide wire for echocardiography guidance is sent along the MPA2 catheter. The head of this special guide wire is expanded into a diamond shape, and the echocardiography can accurately locate its top.

Fix the guide wire, withdraw the MPA2 catheter and the 6F arterial sheath, place the 14F delivery sheath, select the 12 mm × 240 mm BIB balloon and the 3.4 cm CP stent graft, mount the stent on the balloon, and place the stent and balloon along the guide wire into the delivery sheath, the tip of the balloon is closely attached to the bulk of the tip end of the guide wire, and the initial position of the stent is accurately positioned through the expanded guide wire tip end under echocardiography guidance, and the balloon inner capsule and the outer balloon expansion stent are sequentially expanded after the adjustment position is satisfactory. Again, the arterial pressure was 106/64 mmHg in the left upper extremity and 98/52 mmHg in the left lower extremity. Transthoracic echocardiography showed that the position and shape of the stent were good, the patent duct artery was covered by the stent, and the arterial horizontal shunt disappeared. The catheter, guide wire, and arterial sheath were removed and the femoral artery puncture site was sutured with a vascular suturing device.

Treatment efficacy: The patient's symptoms of amaurosis were significantly improved. Echocardiography showed a laminar blood flow in the descending aortic stent with a velocity of blood flow of 2.1 m/s. The procedure time was 30 min; the intraoperative blood loss was 30 mL, and the patient was discharged smoothly 2 days after procedure. The patient was followed up at 1 month after procedure, free of complications.

References

1. Hamdan MA, et al. Endovascular stents for coarctation of the aorta: initial results and intermediate-term follow-up. J Am Coll Cardiol. 2001;38(5):1518–23.
2. Expert committee on congenital heart disease, Chinese association of pediatricians, Chinese medical doctor association. Expert consensus on the treatment of common congenital heart disease in children. Chinese J Pediatr. 2015;53(1):17–24.
3. Cowley CG, et al. Long-term, randomized comparison of balloon angioplasty and surgery for native coarctation of the aorta in childhood. Circulation. 2005;111(25):3453–6.
4. Fish CA. Coarctation of the aorta. J Ky State Med Assoc. 1959;57(6):681–3.

Echocardiography-guided percutaneous intervention for perioperative refinement is essential for early detection of complications and early recovery of patients. Post-procedural treatment focuses on the maintenance of cardiopulmonary function, anticoagulant therapy, etc. Post-procedural complications should be detected and treated in time, and long-term follow-up should be done to objectively evaluate the therapeutic effect. The principle of treatment after echocardiography-guided percutaneous intervention includes early extubation, cardiac function maintenance, and systemic standard management is given special emphisis.

15.1 Key points of Post-procedural Treatment

15.1.1 Protection of Occluder

The occluder should be carefully protected to avoid displacement or shedding.

1. Nursing considerations: The patient should be strictly immobilized and the extremities should be restrained to avoid turning over and other movements in the early postoperative period.
2. Treatment: If the patient's involuntary movement is severe when the patient wakes up, a small dose of sedative drugs as appropriate should be given, with close monitoring of heart rate, blood pressure, central venous pressure, and other hemodynamic parameters to avoid violent fluctuations in the hemodynamics.

15.1.2 Anticoagulation

The aim is to avoid thrombosis associated with metal occluder.

- Anticoagulant regimen: ACT can be monitored after echocardiography-guided percutaneous interventional therapy. When ACT <180 s and the hemodynamics is stable, low-molecular heparin is administered subcutaneously 24 h post-procedure. Special cases may follow the anticoagulant principles in the preceding chapter.
- Monitoring index: Postoperative ACT should be maintained for no less than 200 s. If ACT >300 s, low-dose protamine can be used to neutralize heparin and the application of heparin can be delayed at the same time.
- Aspirin orally: infants, 3–5 mg/(kg·day); and adults, 100–200 mg/day for 6 months.

15.1.3 Cardiac Function Maintenance

The procedure of the occluder implantation may influence cardiac function to some degree.

- Application of vasoactive drugs: In patients with difficulty in occluder placement, long period intracardiac manipulation, significant preoperative pulmonary hypertension or large defects, a small dose of dopamine [2–5 μg/(kg min)], and milrinone should be administered to maintain heart function, support hemodynamics and improve lung compliance in the early postoperative period. If the patient can eat normally after extubation, vasoactive agent administration can be cancelled.
- Other drug applications: Application of corticosteroids to reduce myocardial edema, and use of sodium creatine phosphate to protect myocardium.

15.1.4 Respiratory Management

At present, tracheal intubation is unnecessary in most patients with echocardiography-guided percutaneous intervention. If

X. Pan et al., *Percutaneous and Non-fluoroscopical (PAN) Procedure for Structural Heart Disease*,
https://doi.org/10.1007/978-981-15-2055-6_15

TEE guidance is used, the patients are usually intubated and early extubation is recommended. Respiratory management should be very careful in patients with low weight, young age, or developmental disorder of respiratory tract.

- Prevention and treatment of respiratory tract infections: Postoperative monitoring of body temperature, blood routine, inflammatory indicators, chest X-ray, etc. should be carried out regularly. Antibiotics are given intravenously once half an hour pre-procedure and 6h post-procedure. After procedure, if patients present with cough reflexes and wake up, sputum suctioning should be given carefully to avoid airway spasm. In case of productive cough of purulent yellow sputum, increase the times of sucking as appropriate, and actively retain sputum cultivate to guide antibiotic therapy.
- Extubation timing: Early extubation is encouraged after echocardiography-guided percutaneous intervention to avoid ventilator-associated pneumonia. Extubation usually is performed at 3–5 h post-procedure after sufficient sputum aspiration, when the patient wakes up with stable hemodynamics and satisfactory blood gas results. The key point is to avoid patient agitation during extubation, which could affect occluder stabilization.

15.1.5 Management of Blood Volume

Due to pre-procedural fast and blood loss during procedure, volume depletion should be addressed firstly with crystal and colloid fluid intravenously. After echocardiography-guided percutaneous intervention, shunts from left to right decrease while the volume burden on systemic circulation increases which may lead to transient hypertension. Appropriate diuretics can be used to maintain a negative balance between intake and output volume.

15.2 Post-procedural Complications and Treatment

The main complications after echocardiography-guided percutaneous intervention include occluder displacement or shedding, embolism, etc. Minor complications are mainly arrhythmia. In severe cases, atrioventricular block may occur. Other complications include residual shunt, hemolysis, pericardial effusion, cardiac tamponade, heart rupture, affecting valve movement, and outflow tract obstruction. Early detection and timely treatment of complications are of great importance, and surgical intervention should be applied in time if necessary.

15.2.1 Early Identification

- Arrhythmia is a common complication after echocardiography-guided percutaneous interventional

therapy and is mostly seen in patients with perimembranous ventricular septal defect, which is associated with myocardial edema and transient disruption of conduction system due to procedural stimulation. Frequent episodes of atrial or ventricular premature beats may be the consequence of stimulating the heart with the fallen occluder great attention should be paid to it.

- Inappropriate selection of occluder size or the improper manipulation may result in residual shunt, valvular regurgitation, and outflow tract obstruction. The operator should fully understand the procedure and keep good cooperation with echocardiographer to detect and treat the complications in time.
- For patients with large ASD or ventricular septal defect of subarterial type, the occluder is susceptible to shedding and may result in cardiac tamponade, heart rupture, etc. Clinically, when there are serious fluctuations in hemodynamics, heart sound changes, dynamic changes in electrocardiogram, severe hematuria, changes in hemoglobin, etc., it is necessary to consider the possibility of such malignant events. These severe events can be detected by echocardiography and warrant prompt surgery.
- Insufficient post-procedural anticoagulation may lead to occluder-related thrombosis. The coagulation function and echocardiography should be reviewed in time to confirm the diagnosis.
- We should emphasis on the role of post-procedural auscultation, especially in comparison with the early auscultation of heart sounds, once the obvious murmur or murmur changes are found, the echocardiography should be performed to detect the complications such as occluder displacement and shedding in time, which will be valuable for subsequent treatment.

15.2.2 Timely Treatment and Surgical Intervention

- The arrhythmia and atrioventricular block post echocardiography-guided percutaneous interventional therapy are mostly transient, which should be early treated with corticosteroids and myocardial protection drugs. After treatment, the arrhythmia such as bradycardia or atrioventricular block can be improved. If it persists, implantation of a pacemaker may be necessary.
- The inserted occluder may affect the movement of the valve, block the right ventricular outflow tract or leave residual shunt. The operator should decide whether to switch to the extracorporeal circulation surgery to remove the occluder and perform the traditional repair operation according to the results of echocardiography examination.
- When the hemodynamics fluctuates sharply, and the echocardiography examination indicates the occluder fall off, heart tamponade, heart rupture, or other serious com-

plications, it is necessary to remove the occluder and repair the heart by surgery.

- In the presence of cardiac thrombosis, the intensity and time of anticoagulant therapy should be enhanced, and the therapeutic effect can be judged by combining echocardiographic findings. If necessary, thoracotomy surgery should be performed to remove thrombus.

15.3 Post-procedural Follow-up

To evaluate the long-term effects of echocardiography-guided percutaneous interventional therapy, patients should be followed up at 1, 3, 6, and 12 months after procedure with echocardiography and electrocardiogram.

15.4 Summary

Optimized management, prophylactic therapy, and timely treatment of procedure-related complications post echocardiography-guided percutaneous intervention require close cooperation of the multidisciplinary team to improve the outcomes of this therapy and patient satisfaction.